2011

D0874500

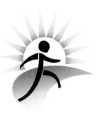

ASTHMA: YOU'RE THE BOSS!

YOU CAN MANAGE IT

Five Steps to Take Charge
of Your Asthma

Gary R. Epler, M.D.

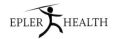
EPLER HEALTH

Epler, Gary R.
Asthma: You're the Boss
You Can Manage It

Library of Congress Cataloging-in-Publication Data: Pending

Library of Congress Control Number: 2011913548
ISBN: 978-0-615-51544-1

The views expressed in this publication are those of the
authors and do not necessarily reflect views of any medical group
or of the staff, officers, or directors of Epler Health, Inc. This publication is
for general informational purposes only, and it is not a substitute for professional
medical advice. This publication does not offer a medical opinion about any
specific facts. Competent medical advice should be sought before any
action is taken in a specific situation by a particular party.

Printed in the United States of America

Other books by Gary Epler:
You're the Boss: Manage Your Disease
BOOP: You're the Boss

This book is dedicated to all individuals throughout the world who have managed their asthma successfully.

Acknowledgments

I would like to thank Dr. Christopher Fanta at Partners Asthma Center in Boston for his innovative development of asthma care for people all over the world and for his phenomenal help writing this book. Thanks also to Glenda Garland for her wonderful writing assistance, to Steve Cumming for his outstanding editing and title development, and to Marian Ferro for her unerring proofreading.

Contents

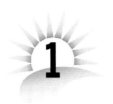

Five Steps Toward Asthma Management

You are in charge of your asthma. You can manage it better than anyone else. Use the five vital steps for success.

- First: Learn everything you can about asthma.
- Second: Understand the diagnostic process.
- Third: Know your treatment options.
- Fourth: Monitor your asthma.
- Fifth: Create a lifetime environment for healing.

This chapter will provide you with the general approach to managing disease. Specifics for managing asthma will be discussed in the chapters that follow.

Let's begin by learning how to take a positive approach to your disease. Traditionally, people see the doctor, have tests and treatment, and return to the doctor. This is too passive. Without your active participation, this approach can lead to diagnostic confusion, muddled treatment, and sporadically uncontrolled disease. The successful approach is to actively take charge and manage your disease.

———

Andy was a busy man. He was in his mid-30s and had a successful business, which kept him active and excited about each day. He suddenly found himself in the emergency room unable to breathe, and he was angry. The doctors told him he had an asthma attack, and he didn't want to hear about it.

Why did he have asthma? He remembered that someone in his family had used an inhaler when he was young, but that was a long time ago. Besides, he'd never been sick. "This isn't asthma," he told himself. "These doctors don't know what they're talking about."

Andy was given two nebulizer treatments and was discharged. He was instructed as to how to use an inhaler, but he didn't pay attention.

A few days later, Andy felt tightness in his chest and began wheezing. He tried the inhaler but didn't know how to use it properly so his wheezing worsened. He returned to the ER and once again received treatment to stop the attack. He became frustrated and angrier. "Why can't the doctors make this go away?" he thought. "I have to get to work."

Andy had more asthma attacks and was instructed in using a new preventive medicine inhaler that contained corticosteroid – a powerful anti-inflammatory agent.

He was also told about asthma as inflammation of the airways that can be triggered by respiratory infections and allergies. Several tests were recommended in an attempt to determine the type of asthma that afflicted him. Again, he failed to pay attention. This would go away, he thought.

Andy became so confused about which inhaler to use that he stopped using both of them. As expected, he once again returned to the ER because of severe wheezing. This time, he was given the corticosteroid medicine intravenously and had to stay in the overnight observation unit.

At discharge, he was given prednisone, an oral form of corticosteroid medication, to take on a tapering dose during the week.

These steroid tablets were so good that Andy told himself he could take them instead of listening to the doctors talk on and on about the types of asthma and using the preventive inhalers. This worked great for him – he felt some chest tightness, took a few prednisone tablets, and went to work. Yet Andy had failed to learn anything about the adverse reactions associated with taking prednisone long-term. He quickly found out. Andy gained weight. His face became chubby. His blood sugar level increased, and he used an entire canister of the bronchodilator inhaler every few days to control his wheezing.

His asthma was way out of control. He had a severe attack and ended up in the hospital's intensive care unit.

Andy's experience is not the way to manage asthma.

Sue's story is different. She learned how to manage her asthma successfully.

———

Sue was in her late 20s and had a successful job. Suddenly and unexpectedly, she had an asthma attack and was treated in the emergency room.

She was frightened and blamed herself at first, but she realized that this attitude did more harm than good. Instead she told herself that she could manage the situation.

Sue began to learn about asthma from the doctors and nurses, and she explored the internet. She learned that she should find out what type of asthma she had and underwent diagnostic studies as directed by her doctor.

She found out that she had a special type called exercise-induced asthma. Then she learned about the treatment options.

For this type of asthma, a bronchodilator inhaler can be helpful, especially before exercise. Asthma causes constriction of the airways, and this type of inhaler dilates or enlarges the airways by inducing relaxation of the small circular muscles that surround the airways. Sue used the inhaler before her exercise session and had a seven-minute warm-up. Soon she was able to exercise without difficulty.

Sue also had typical asthma that was controlled by an anti-inflammatory inhaler. She learned that in addition to constricted airway openings, people with asthma have inflammation of the airways, so an anti-inflammatory medication referred to as corticosteroid was helpful to prevent attacks. She started using a corticosteroid inhaler once in the morning and had no future serious attacks.

Sue learned her asthma triggers in addition to exercise and avoided them. She learned to monitor her symptoms so that she could know when to use the bronchodilator inhaler. She also developed a routine exercise program, reviewed her nutritional program, and developed a good sleeping pattern.

She managed the asthma so well that she was able to do everything she wanted professionally and socially. Her asthma no longer was an activity-limiting disease. It had been melded into her life as a routine.

———

Andy did everything wrong. He was angry and refused to learn about asthma. He failed to obtain diagnostic testing that would determine the type of asthma he had. He refused to use the corticosteroid inhaler regularly. He used only his rescue inhaler, and didn't learn how to use it properly. He spent too much of his time in the emergency room. He lost time at work and he was frequently sick. He couldn't participate in sports or social events. He developed serious side effects from prednisone and was headed for prolonged hospitalizations with potential life-threatening complications.

Sue did everything right. She asked questions. She learned about asthma and found out what type of asthma she had. She understood when to use the rescue inhaler and the benefits of using the prevention inhaler every day. She developed an exercise program, a good nutrition program, and a healthy sleep schedule. She took charge. She managed her asthma and did not allow it to interfere with her life. She was able to work successfully, participate in all types of sports, and had an active social life.

So, how do you take charge of your asthma?

Follow the five vital steps.

Begin with the first one: **Learn everything you can about asthma.**

Ask your doctor about asthma and obtain information from the clinic. Ask the nurse educators – they can be unlimited sources of information and help you learn to manage your asthma. Read reports. Read scientific studies. Explore the internet to discover the best websites for you. Visit social media sites and join a session about asthma. You'll find people who have similar questions and concerns. They'll be just like you, and you'll find out how they managed their asthma.

New solutions to asthma problems and new ways to manage asthma are being developed through the global internet community.

After you've learned about asthma, follow the second step: **Understand the diagnostic process.**

A diagnosis has three components that include an organized series of questions, a physical examination, and a sequential group of diagnostic tests and procedures. The first two components require your close attention. It's the third that requires your active participation so that you can make decisions that are best for you.

For asthma, you'll be asked about your wheezing. When did it start? What triggers the wheezing? You'll be asked about non-respiratory symptoms and chronic conditions you might have. You'll be asked about lung diseases that may occur in your family. You'll be asked about allergies to food, pollen or dust, and about adverse drug reactions. You'll be asked about your past respiratory conditions, and occupational and environmental exposures.

During the physical examination, your doctor will take your vital signs and perform an oxygen saturation test. Your lungs will be examined for wheezing.

Ask questions during the sequential group of diagnostic tests and procedures. Nonspecific random testing that searches for a nonspecific diagnosis often leads to confusion, a poor diagnostic yield, and wasted time. So ask, what will this test show? Is there a wide range of normal findings? Do the findings correlate with the disease process? What are the benefits of the diagnostic tests? What are the risks of the procedures? What are the alternatives?

Determine the specific reason for the test, and if it makes sense to you, proceed with it.

_____

Let's hear about Pete. He gradually developed a wheezing sound when he exhaled, and especially after exertion. It bothered him enough to go to the doctor.

"You might have asthma," the doctor said.

"I've never had asthma before," Pete said. "No one in the family has asthma. Why would I have asthma now?"

"Let's first do some tests to make sure it's asthma," the doctor said.

Pete had pulmonary function tests that showed no change after receiving a bronchodilator inhalation.

"That's unusual," the doctor said. "For people with asthma, there is often a 15% to 20% increase in the forced expired volume in one second – the FEV_1 test."

"Does that mean I don't have asthma?" Pete asked.

"Maybe," the doctor said. "I noticed part of your flow-volume curve was flattened, which suggests there may be an obstruction in your airway. Let's obtain a chest computer scan, or computed tomography (CT), to see if something shows up."

After the test, the doctor reviewed the scan with Pete. "Look at the center of the trachea. That's this dark, oval-shaped shadow," the doctor said. "There appears to be a gray lobular structure where it shouldn't be."

"You're scaring me, Doc," Pete said. "What is it? Is it a cancer?"

"We can't tell by looking at the scan. We need to do a bronchoscopy."

"What's that?" Pete asked.

"A small-diameter tube with a lighted tip is inserted through your nose to search for that shadow we saw on the x-ray to find out what it is. If it's a polyp with an attached stalk, it can be snared and removed."

"That sounds good to me, but what are the risks of the bronchoscopy?" Pete asked.

"In this situation they're minimal. You're healthy and have no underlying lung disease or any other health problems, and you're not allergic to the lidocaine that's used for a local anesthetic. However, bleeding may occur, that in a rare situation may be difficult to control, requiring surgical intervention."

"What are the alternatives?"

"You can do nothing and continue observation," the doctor said. "If this is a benign tumor, it will continue to grow, eventually plugging the airway, and if it's a cancer, it will spread to other organs."

"That doesn't sound good to me. The benefits definitely seem to outweigh the risks," Pete said. "Let's go forward with the bronchoscopy."

Pete had the procedure without complications or adverse reactions. His doctor found an adenoma, which is a benign tumor that was attached to the tracheal wall by a stalk, and easily snared by the bronchoscopist and removed. Pete had no recurrence.

———

Pete discovered that "all that wheezes might not be asthma." It's rare, but it happens. Instead of jumping to conclusions, however, at each step

Pete asked questions until he understood the answers. He understood the benefits, the risks, and the alternatives for the diagnostic procedure. Use the second step – understand the diagnostic process.

Now that you have followed the initial two steps for asthma management, let's discuss the third one: **Know everything you can about your treatment options.**

Every situation is unique, and one of the options is going to be best for you.

Ask questions about the effectiveness and risks of the various treatments. Some people like to find out about statistics. What are the alternatives? What are the benefits and side effects of the alternative treatments?

It's important to understand the natural history of asthma. What happens if you decide not to have treatment? The answer will allow you to know what to expect and to be in control of the situation. It will also give you a benchmark to monitor your treatment plan. Learn and understand all of the available information about the benefits and risks of the treatment options.

You now understand the diagnostic process and the treatment options. The next step is to follow the fourth vital rule of management: **Monitor your asthma.**

Monitoring is especially important for asthma because an attack can begin quietly without you being aware of it, and it's at this stage that you could prevent a disabling attack.

It's helpful to be aware of your triggers, and to be on the lookout for them, and to connect them to the early sensation of chest discomfort or tightness in the chest. These triggers include respiratory infections, allergens such as pollen or animal dander, cold air, and exercise.

Ask yourself three questions. Am I better? If so, stay the course. Am I the same? If so, give it time and re-evaluate in a few hours. Am I worse? It may be time to see your doctor, and if it's really worse, visit the emergency room.

The monitoring system can be as simple as reviewing the situation in your mind, or better yet, entering symptoms such as chest tightness, wheezing, shortness of breath, or a cough into the computer, and creating a graphic image of the disease so that you'll have a color-coded visualization of its clinical course. The images will help show you the sequence of symptoms, triggering events, and when a rescue inhaler is needed. With this information, you can choose the course of action that's best for you.

Peak-flow monitoring can be helpful for some people with asthma.

To monitor peak flow, obtain a peak-flow meter, blow into the device, and record the value. This will establish a baseline and monitor for potential episodes of asthma attacks. Recording activities during peak-flow monitoring can also detect asthma triggers.

The monitoring system can be useful in managing your asthma and preventing dangerous attacks that might send you to the hospital.

———

Amanda's story illustrates the usefulness of monitoring asthma.

She was coaching her child's soccer team and wanted to avoid an asthma attack during practices or games. She realized that if she could develop a good monitoring system, use the corticosteroid inhaler, and know when to use the rescue inhaler, she could control her asthma.

"I need a monitoring system," Amanda told her asthma nurse.

"That's a great idea," the nurse said. "Let's put one together for you. What are your asthma triggers?"

"Let's see, they include freshly mowed grass and pollen in the fall," Amanda said.

"Hmm. That could be difficult for a soccer coach, but you'll be surprised by what we can do," the nurse said. "You can use the bronchodilator inhaler beforehand if you are going to be in a trigger zone. Second, you need to monitor your feelings and symptoms. Check in with yourself periodically. Compared to a while ago, how are you feeling – any chest discomfort, chest tightness, wheezing, or cough? Am I better? Am I the same? Am I worse? If worse, you need to pay close attention and may need to use your rescue inhaler."

"That sounds good to me," Amanda said. "I can do that without interfering with my coaching."

"To really do it right," the nurse said, "you need to monitor your peak flow."

"That sounds like a ton of work and way too much for me," Amanda said. "I'm too busy to even try it."

"Yes, it's work and time-consuming in the beginning," the nurse replied, "but you get used to it, and it will be worth it because you'll find out what your baseline value is, find out if you have other triggers; and most importantly, over time, it has the subtle but powerful effect of smoothing out the course of your asthma, eliminating the peaks and valleys."

Amanda quickly learned how to use the peak flow monitor. She followed the monitoring steps and even marked the events on her computer. It paid off. She was amazed at how well she did and how well-controlled her asthma became over time. She continued her daily corticosteroid inhaler and rarely needed her bronchodilator rescue inhaler. During practices and Saturday morning games, Amanda found herself enjoying every minute and not even thinking about her asthma.

———

You've reached the final process for managing your asthma. Use the fifth vital step: **Create a healing environment**.

Let's start with the traditional components: exercise, nutrition and sleep.

Exercise can provide phenomenal benefits in the management of asthma. It improves muscle conditioning, allowing you to do more things without symptoms. It makes you feel good, and importantly, it has a leveling effect by smoothing out the ups and downs of asthma.

A pulmonary rehabilitation program is a great place to start. The program will teach you about your asthma and help you design a weekly exercise program that you can do in your home or at any workout facility. Rehabilitation professionals can create an exercise that is best for your asthma. Remember to add strength training as part of your exercise program because it is helpful for maintaining lean-body mass.

Eating the highest quality of foods in the right amount at the right time will provide positive energy to help you manage your asthma. Advice on how and what to eat seemingly changes every day. People can become overwhelmed and confused with so much conflicting scientific and anecdotal information. But it's important to understand everything possible about nutrition. Read a book, listen to a CD, or go the American Dietetic Association website. Nutritional management is an important part of creating a healing environment.

Meeting with a professional nutritionist can be useful because huge advances have been made in understanding the complexities of the body's metabolism. Nutritionists can design a program specifically for you with the best types and quantities of foods. You'll be able to determine a healthy weight for you, percentage of body fat, the number of calories for your body type, and the amount of water you need each day.

Sleep is the third potent traditional tool used to create an environment in which to heal and stay healthy. After years of study, eight hours of sleep appears to be a requirement for a healthy life for the majority of people. Most people just don't get enough sleep.

Take the five-minute sleep test. Sit in a chair in a quiet room. If you fall asleep within five minutes, you flunk the test. This might be an isolated result, but it also might mean that you are chronically sleep-deprived, which causes neural behavioral changes and cardiovascular complications.

A healthy sleep-hygiene program consists of not allowing yourself to fall asleep watching television before you go to bed, not eating or eating lightly within at least three hours before you go to sleep, and going to bed and awakening at regular times.

Now that you've learned the three traditional methods for creating a healing environment, use your mind and the power of your thoughts. Your body has an almost unlimited ability to heal itself and control disease. You have to know how to let this happen, as the ability may be dormant or blunted by the intensity of daily life.

First, use a positive approach as you deal with your asthma, as Sue did. Amanda did too. She had a great attitude. She wanted to coach soccer and enjoy it, and she wanted to manage her asthma, and she did. Say to yourself that you can manage your asthma. Have overpowering confidence in yourself and your ability to manage it. You will have more energy, follow the medication schedule, and take control.

Second, use visualization. Visualize healthy airways. Every cell in your body is continuously replaced, some every few minutes and others every few weeks or months. Visualize healthy, strong cells replacing the inflamed or dysfunctional cells. Begin by replacing a few cells, but think big and ultimately visualize replacing millions. You can use this visualization process anytime you wish, and you can monitor the process with your disease-monitoring system.

Third, have compassion for your lungs. They're functionally perfect. The asthma is causing the dysfunction, and the inflamed cells can be replaced with healthy cells.

Fourth, used controlled breathing. During a time when you're not having an asthma attack, breathe in fully, filling your lungs with air and exhaling an equal amount. Repeat this several times until you have a feeling of calm. If you wish, you can breathe in healthy energy and exhale neutralized energy. You also can take big chest breaths during exercise to spread oxygen and energy throughout your body.

Take belly breaths to relieve stress. Place your hand on your abdomen and breathe in, moving your hand up. Take three or four breaths, they can have an amazingly calming effect. If you are stressed while eating a meal, take these belly breaths before you begin. They will be calming and can even improve digestion.

Incidentally, traditional yoga was based on breathing, and the right yoga instructor and class can be helpful to your asthma management.

Fifth, be persistent, as these methods are subtle, requiring repetition and time, sometimes weeks or months. Our bodies have an endless energy-based system that can be used to create powerful changes to improve our lives.

In the next chapters, each of the five steps will be discussed in detail as you learn how to manage your asthma.

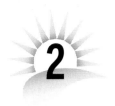

What's Asthma?
Inflamed Airways and Bronchospasm

Physicians have recognized the symptoms of asthma for thousands of years. Ancient Egyptian and Greek doctors described asthmatic patients. The word asthma is from the Greek language, and means to pant or to breathe hard.

We currently define asthma in terms of its symptoms, because there is no blood test or measurement or biomarker that we can point to and say, "Oh yes, that's asthma."

Asthma is inflammation of the airways and bronchospasm. The inflammation occurs in the bronchial airways, which are the slender tubes that branch out from your trachea, or windpipe. Bronchospasm is the periodic contraction of the smooth, circular muscles around the bronchial airways. This can quickly narrow your airways and keep them that way for seconds to minutes.

The airway inflammation plugs up the bronchial airways with congestion, and the bronchospasm further decreases the amount of air you can draw into the lungs. These two features account for the typical symptoms of asthma, such as wheezing, coughing, and chest tightness, which is like someone squeezing you with a bear hug.

The symptoms come and go. They can vary in intensity and how symptoms present themselves, and their effects can be reversed. But a person who has asthma always has asthma, even if symptoms are not there on a given day. Asthma is a chronic condition with intermittent symptoms. Think of it as a vulnerability to inflammation and bronchospasm, as if your bronchial airways are waiting to be provoked. To manage your asthma successfully, you need to address both these underlying features. You need to manage the airway inflammation and the bronchospasm.

––––

Let's talk about Ben. He knew he had asthma. He'd known for years. He carried an albuterol inhaler, a bronchodilator, and used it whenever he felt his chest tighten or started to wheeze. This happened perhaps once a week or every other week. But lately he had been waking up at night coughing, and using the inhaler much more frequently.

"Why is this happening?" he asked himself. "Why does it feel like my asthma is getting worse?"

"So far," his doctor said, "we've been able to treat your asthma with just the bronchodilator that controls the airway muscle spasm.

"But, now, it sounds like we need to treat the underlying inflammation part of your asthma. Let's get you started on an inhaled steroid. They're safe, because they target the bronchial airways and don't go much farther into the body."

Ben began taking a daily, low-dose, inhaled steroid, and soon he needed his bronchodilator only about once a month. By learning more about both features of asthma – inflammation and bronchospasm – Ben learned how to successfully manage his asthma.

––––

About 8% of people in the United States have asthma. That's 25 million people, and the worldwide estimate is 300 million people.

The cause of the underlying vulnerability is not known. Research has focused on the immune system cells. The bronchial airways of people with asthma often have eosinophils, which are white blood cells with red granules associated with allergies, and mast cells, which are large tissue cells related to asthma. Eosinophils and mast cells show up in great numbers during allergic reactions in other tissues. They're present in the eyes when someone has itchy eyes or in the nose when someone has a watery nose due to hay fever or high pollen levels. Therefore, the eosinophils and mast cells in the bronchial airways may be one allergic response among a constellation of other allergic responses.

The allergic responses result as our immune system cells respond to a foreign substance. Our genes contain the codes to create our immune system, which means that we may inherit our allergic sensitivities from our parents, and for asthma, it appears to be more commonly inherited from our mothers. If your mother has asthma, you might too. It is not always inherited. For example, asthma develops in about one-third of identical twins who have mothers with asthma. It's not just genetics. How you interact with your environment also matters.

Extensive research is has been undertaken to identify the genetics behind the immune system and understand the interaction of environmental factors with the genetic code. For example, why do some people develop eye and nose allergies but not bronchial airways allergies?

Asthma is on the rise in Westernized countries, especially in the cities. Air pollution alone doesn't account for this increase. Some of the increase may be due to the sedentary urban lifestyle. Also, the frequency of asthma and allergies appears to be related to people's weight – the higher the weight, the higher the frequency of asthma.

Other factors that might cause the increase in asthma include the greater concentration of indoor allergens, as people try to restrict the airflow in and out of their houses to conserve energy and to lower heating and cooling costs.

Despite not knowing the underlying causes, doctors recognize different types of asthma. As we've already learned from Andy, Sue, Pete, Amanda, and Ben, asthma symptoms can vary greatly, in kind and in severity. Before we learn about the specific types, let's hear about Billy Norton's story.

———

Billy was healthy but struggling to accomplish his goals. He wanted to go to law school but was frustrated by trying to study for the entrance examination. He needed a high score to get into a prestigious law school. Several years after graduating from college, he was working two full-time jobs with long hours and low pay as he tried to pay off college loans and study for the law exam late at night.

Suddenly, he developed wheezing and shortness of breath.

"What's going on? I don't need this?" he thought.

He didn't have much time to dwell on his problem because his breathing became so labored that he had to get to the hospital emergency room as fast as he could.

The triage nurse rushed him to the acute care ER room and summoned the doctor.

"You're probably having an asthma attack," Dr. Gooden said. "Your airways are clamped shut and we need to give you a breathing treatment to open them up. We'll also start intravenous fluid and give you additional bronchodilator medicine."

"I can't breathe," Billy said, on the verge of panic.

"It's hard to believe at this time, but you have plenty of oxygen," the doctor assured him. "You need to know that you have enough oxygen so you can concentrate on your breathing. Try to slow it down. Breathe through your nose, and out through your mouth. Put your hand on your stomach and feel the tightness as you breathe out."

"I can't do it, I can't," Billy shrieked, breathing so fast that he couldn't talk in a complete sentence and couldn't listen to the doctor.

"Yes, you can," Dr. Gooden said in a soft, firm voice. "Your oxygen level is good and not faltering. Try to slow down your breathing anyway you can."

"I'm-m-m trying," Billy said with a stammer. "My chest is so tight I can't breathe."

The doctor could hear a high-pitched wheeze during each breath. "Keep trying. The medicine will begin to work in a few breaths."

Billy was fighting for each breath, but realized he could slow his breathing.

"Now, breathe in through your nose and out your mouth," the doctor reminded Billy.

"I'm trying," Billy said, continuing to struggle.

Billy had been treated with a nebulizer aerosol and fluids from an intravenous catheter. His vital signs were taken and showed a good blood pressure, but he had a rapid pulse rate and extremely rapid respiratory rate. His temperature was normal, and his oxygen saturation value was normal despite his shallow, ineffective breaths.

"It's working. I'm beginning to breathe again," Billy said, now more calmly.

"Good, let's find out what happened," the doctor said.

———

Billy was at the first step. He was going to learn about asthma and had started the process to learn much more. For the next step, he was going to understand the diagnostic process.

Next, we'll learn about the different types of asthma.

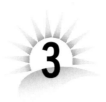

Which of the Types of Asthma Do You Have?

Part of successfully managing asthma involves knowing what type of asthma you have.

Childhood Asthma

Most asthma develops during childhood beginning between ages five and seven. Among children with asthma, about 80% have allergies, which can show up not only as red eyes and watery noses, but as eczema, which causes red, scaly rashes on the skin. Depending on a child's age, symptoms of asthma may include coughing, gasping, not wanting to eat or exercise, chest tightness, wheezing with respiratory infections, and, especially, wheezing when the child does not have a respiratory infection.

———

When Wendy was three, her mother, Anne, noticed that Wendy was not shaking off the cold she'd contracted a few weeks ago. The little girl was coughing frequently, and her cough was waking her up from naps and at night.

Anne noticed that Wendy had little interest it in going to the park and climbing on the playground structures. Then, on a sunny spring day when Wendy was running around at the park, her breath made a whistling noise. She was wheezing.

Anne took Wendy to her pediatrician.

"Does Wendy show any signs of allergies like hay fever or eczema," the doctor asked. "Do you or your husband have allergies or asthma?"

"I have some mild hay fever during the spring and fall seasons with the sniffles, but nothing else," Anne said. "Wendy doesn't appear to have sign of allergies."

"She probably has reactive airway disorder," Wendy's doctor said. "She looks great. There is no wheezing now. Let's monitor the situation."

Anne researched reactive airway disorder at home. She learned that since signs of asthma are not always clear-cut in children and asthma tests may be inconclusive in children under six years old, many pediatricians make the more cautious diagnosis of reactive airway disorder, ARD, which is a term used to describe wheezing or breathing difficulties often associated with mild respiratory infections or dust, without identifying its specific cause.

Several months later, Wendy again began cough and wheezing.

"Is anything different this time?" the pediatrician asked.

"I don't think so," Anne said. "She just started wheezing again."

"Has she developed any skin allergies?" the doctor asked.

"Oh, you asked me that before," Anne said. "And, we noticed that Wendy developed some eczema on her arms."

"That's often a sign of allergies," the pediatrician said. "Did she have any asthma triggers?"

"I'm not sure there's a connection, but we had new carpet installed just before she developed wheezing."

"Yes, there are chemicals in new carpets that may cause irritation in people with asthma," the pediatrician said. "This was recognized several years ago, and most of the irritant chemicals have been removed, but sometimes the dust from removing the old carpet can cause an asthma flare-up."

"That was likely the problem," Anne said. "It was really dusty."

"This time I'll give you a bronchodilator inhaler for Wendy," the pediatrician said. "Call me during the next two or three days to let me know if it's helping her."

When Anne reported that it had, the pediatrician said. "Wendy probably has asthma. Let's talk and figure out a plan to make sure we manage it correctly."

Adult-Onset Asthma

Asthma may develop at any age. Up to one-third of people with asthma have their first attack after age 30. Most people who develop asthma as an adult, however, probably had a mild form as children that faded during adolescence.

The exact relationship between hormones and asthma isn't clear, although there might be some connection with estrogen. A woman who has asthma can show dramatically different symptoms during pregnancy. Some women show more symptoms around their periods, and some postmenopausal women who take estrogen supplements have a slightly higher risk of developing asthma.

People with allergies who did not have asthma as children can develop asthma as adults. Some viral infections might trigger an unusual form of bronchial airway inflammation that results in underlying twitchiness of the airways, producing asthma. Smokers also might develop asthma as adults because tobacco smoke alters the surface of bronchial airways and makes them hypersensitive.

————

Scott took up smoking in college and developed a thick cough and morning phlegm. As he was smoking one day, he started wheezing and feeling like his roommate, a wrestler, had him in a serious chest hold.

"I can't breathe," he gasped.

"Let's go!" his roommate exclaimed. "I'm taking you to the campus ER."

"You're having an asthma attack," the doctor said, as the nurse administered a hand-held nebulizer bronchodilator treatment to relax his bronchial airways.

"Asthma!" Scott said with astonishment. "I don't have asthma. My cousin, who's seven, has asthma. She's had it since she was two. You're supposed to get it when you're a kid. I'm safe."

"Do you smoke?" his doctor asked.

"Yes, but only a pack a day," Scott said with some guilt.

"The cigarette smoke has caused inflammation in your bronchial airways," the doctor said. "These are the medium-to-large, branching airways leading into your lungs. That's what caused your cough and the congestion in your chest. You're one of those people whose lungs just can't handle the cigarette smoke."

"You mean I have to quit?" Scott asked.

"Yes, you must quit," the doctor said. "I'll give you inhalers to control the wheezing and inflammation, but it will be difficult to control your asthma with continual irritation and inflammation from the cigarette smoke."

"Sounds like I will have to. I don't want that attack to happen again."

"You and me both," his roommate joined in.

Aspirin-Induced Asthma

A small segment of people, about 5%, who have adult-onset asthma will also develop a sensitivity to aspirin and all other NSAIDs, or non-steroidal anti-inflammatory drugs like ibuprofen such as Advil® and Motrin® or naproxen sodium such as Aleve®. These people also tend to have intermittent chest congestion and sinusitis, and they often have nasal polyps, which are grape-like growths in the nose.

———

Maggie was a successful self-employed entrepreneur who had just celebrated her 32nd birthday.

"I feel like I have a cold that won't seem to go away," she told Dr. Martin Lewis.

"You may have a bacterial bronchitis, so I'll give you an antibiotic pack," Dr. Lewis said.

The bronchitis resolved with the antibiotic. Several weeks passed. The congestion and cough recurred and became uncomfortable, especially whenever Maggie contracted a cold. She also developed wheezing with the cold. After a year Dr. Lewis diagnosed her with asthma. She learned everything she could about asthma and learned about inhalers and medicines. She managed her asthma extremely well, and her business boomed.

Suddenly the following year, "I can't breathe," she gasped as the ER doctor inserted the intravenous catheter. "I'm having an asthma attack!" she exclaimed.

Maggie was admitted for observation and the asthma was quickly stabilized.

"What triggered the attack?" Dr. Lewis asked her as he stopped by to see her during his hospital rounds.

"I'm not sure," a puzzled Maggie answered. "I didn't have a cold or an infection. I don't think I had any allergy exposures, and I didn't have any chemical exposures.

I had a headache and took an aspirin, but that can't be related," Maggie continued.

"You'd be surprised," Dr. Lewis said. "Some people with asthma can be very sensitive to aspirin and its counterparts. You have aspirin-induced asthma, and I would suggest that you use acetaminophen [Tylenol®] for pain.

A year later Maggie found out that she needed to have two of her remaining wisdom teeth removed. If that wasn't challenge enough, her dentist prescribed ibuprofen for the pain.

"I don't think I can take that," she told the dentist. "I have aspirin-sensitive asthma."

"It'll be fine," her dentist said.

But Maggie wasn't convinced. When she went to purchase the medicine, she asked the pharmacist if she could take the ibuprofen.

"Oh, no," the pharmacist said. "You shouldn't take ibuprofen or similar anti-inflammatory medicines if you have aspirin-sensitive asthma. Here's a list of what you should avoid. Talk to your dentist about other pain-relief options."

Allergy Asthma

This type of asthma occurs when asthma symptoms develop from exposure to specific allergenic triggers, which include animal dander, molds and pollen as well as the protein material from cockroaches, mouse feces and dust mites.

———

Every Friday night Aidan went to his friend Bill's house to play poker. But during a stretch of three Fridays, by the time he arrived at home, he'd feel as if someone was squeezing his chest with a rubber band, and he had to use his inhaler for relief. He couldn't figure out what was causing it because his friend was a neatnik and no one smoked cigarettes. Nothing in Bill's house had ever bothered Aiden before.

On the fourth Friday night, a black-and-white cat jumped onto the green, baize-covered poker table and then sauntered away.

"Hey," Bill said, "Pockets finally came out of his hiding place. He's my girlfriend's cat, and I've been babysitting while she's been out of the country. I thought he'd hide under the upstairs dresser until she comes home."

"Cute cat," Aiden said, as and thought to himself, "*Now I know what's triggering my asthma.*"

Exercise-Induced Asthma

Like allergy asthma, other types of asthma have specific triggers. For some people, like Sue, whom we met in the first chapter, exercise is the only thing that triggers her asthma. Sue had her attack a few minutes after she stopped exercising, which may happen to some people; to others, chest tightness and wheezing can occur within a few moments while running after a bus on a cold morning. Exercise causes you to breathe more, and exercise, especially on cold, dry days, can trigger bronchospasm. People who have these reactions do have asthma, and it is referred to as "exercised-induced bronchoconstriction" because the bronchospasm, rather than underlying inflammation and congestion, drives symptoms for these people.

Occupational Asthma

Some people may develop asthma from exposures at work and others may develop asthma from exposures while doing their hobbies such as making pottery or sculpting at home. Work-related asthma is defined as asthma that is caused, or triggered, by an inhalation exposure in the workplace. Work-exacerbated asthma is defined as asthma triggered by various work-related factors in people who have pre-existing asthma.

There are two types of occupational asthma. The first is called sensitizer-induced occupational asthma and is defined as new-onset asthma induced by sensitization to a specific substance at work. This means that a person becomes allergic to the substance or chemical. It usually takes several weeks or months to develop the sensitivity. Examples include carpenters who work with red cedar shingles or bakers who use different types of flour. Occupational asthma develops from specific substances, and once it's established, a small exposure to the specific substance will trigger an asthma attack. For example, a baker may develop asthma sensitivity to rye flour but not to wheat flour. Workers may develop sensitivity to unusual exposures such as castor bean dust or saltwater king crab. Some chemicals such as isocyanates and the epoxies can cause sensitizing asthma.

The second is called irritant-induced occupational asthma and is defined as new-onset asthma or the recurrence of past asthma induced by exposure to an inhaled irritant at work and meeting criteria of reactive airways dysfunction syndrome, or RADS. This type of occupational asthma usually occurs from a one-time exposure to a large volume of an irritant chemical such as ammonia or chlorine, often from an accidental chemical leak or explosion.

———

Now that we've discussed the different types of asthma, we'll explore the diagnostic process for asthma. This will help you learn how to manage your asthma successfully.

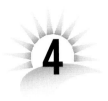

Diagnosing Your Asthma:
Questions, Examination, Tests

The diagnostic process has three components: a group of questions, a physical examination, and a series of diagnostic tests. The first two components require your close attention. It's the third that requires your active participation so that you can make decisions that are best for you.

After meeting your physician, you will be asked about the onset of your asthma. When did it start? Did it start with the flu or a cold? Did it start with exposure to pollen or other allergens?

You'll be asked the five questions about your lungs. Do you have a cough, phlegm, wheezing, shortness of breath, or do you cough up blood?

If you have a cough, when did it begin? Does it occur every day? Does it occur at night? Coughing means irritation of the airways, which might also mean airway inflammation or abnormalities in the lungs. The cough may be due to inflammation in the moderate-to-large airways called bronchi or the small ones called bronchioles. Other causes of airway inflammation can include a postnasal drip, stomach acid from esophageal reflux that irritates the airways, or tumors.

You'll be asked about phlegm or sputum production. Is there phlegm with the cough? When does it occur – in the morning, throughout the day, or in the evening? How much – a teaspoon or a half-cup?

Millions of glands in the airways produce mucus and defensive substances to keep the airways moist and to protect against disease, and mucus production occurs constantly at an undetectable level. Inflammation, however, will cause an increase in mucus and phlegm. If an infection is causing the inflammation, the mucus will be yellow and green in color. You might need antibiotics. Sometimes, yellow phlegm may be produced in a severe asthma attack from a huge number of white blood cells called eosinophils that contain red granules.

Wheezing, or a whistling sound during an expiratory breath, is the important symptom for asthma. It's the most common symptom. When does the wheezing occur – in the morning or at night? If you have a cough, does the wheezing occur before or after the cough? What triggers the wheezing? It's helpful to identify the triggers because knowing these "asthma triggers" can alert you to an expected asthma attack early so it can be prevented. How intense is the wheezing? Is it constant or intermittent?

Wheezing indicates bronchospasm, which as noted in a previous chapter, is the constriction of the smooth circular muscles that surround the airways in the lungs. Usually these muscles give the airways shape and prevent them from collapsing, but during bronchospasm, the narrowed airways create a high-pitched wheezing sound when you exhale. In severe situations, the wheezing occurs also when you inhale.

The fourth question is about shortness of breath. Is there shortness of breath or breathlessness with certain activities? How severe is the shortness of breath? The severity can be graded on a scale of one to four. In grade one, a person is out of breath during exertional activities. In grade two, shortness of breath can occur climbing a flight of stairs. In grade three, a person has shortness of breath walking on level ground for less than 100 yards. In severe grade four, a person has shortness of breath performing routine activities such as talking or dressing.

Shortness of breath means a major portion of the lung is involved. So many airways are constricted that the lungs cannot receive enough oxygen. Other causes of shortness of breath include lungs that are filled with infection-related pneumonia or diffuse inflammation, or weakened heart or diaphragm.

The fifth respiratory question is about blood in the sputum, which may be caused by severe inflammation of the airways from an infection-related bronchitis or from inflammation in the lungs related to pneumonia. Blood in the phlegm may be due to a tumor in the airways or the lungs. In an unusual situation, a blood clot in the lungs in the form of a pulmonary embolism can cause blood in sputum.

You'll be asked about non-respiratory symptoms such as fever, chills, muscle and joint pains, loss of appetite, and weight loss or night sweats to find out whether the wheezing may be caused by an underlying condition in the lungs, or even outside of the lungs.

Next, you'll be asked about smoking. Did you ever smoke? If you did, when did you start? How many cigarettes did you smoke per day? When did you stop? Have you smoked cigars or pipes? Do you chew tobacco or use snuff? You'll be asked whether you drink alcohol, and if so, what types, how much, and how frequently?

You'll be asked about lung diseases that may occur in your family such as asthma, allergies, bronchitis, emphysema, lung fibrosis or scarring, lung cancer, or tuberculosis. This information is helpful in determining whether your asthma has a family connection.

You'll be asked similar questions about your past respiratory conditions such as whether you've had bronchitis, pneumonia or pleurisy. Do you develop head colds or chest colds? Have you had sinus infections? Have you had a postnasal drip, which can be a cause of cough and can cause wheezing? You'll especially be asked about allergies to food, pollen or dust. Do you develop watery eyes, a rash, or wheezing from these allergies? Are the symptoms seasonal?

You'll be asked about adverse drug reactions. Are you allergic to any medications? If so, did you develop a rash, nausea, or dizziness from a particular medication? How severe was the reaction? Some symptoms may be an allergy to the medicine while others may be from the effects of a dosage that's too high for you.

Several non-pulmonary questions will be asked. Do you have any medical conditions such as diabetes, high blood pressure, heart disease, stomach ulcers and importantly, gastroesophageal reflux disease, or GERD, as this condition can cause coughing or wheezing.

Do you have heart disease, chronic hepatitis, kidney disease, rheumatological or immunological disorders, seizures or neurological conditions, or cancer? This information is helpful in determining whether the asthma is associated with an underlying medical condition. You'll also be asked about past surgical procedures.

Each organ system will be reviewed. Have you had any skin rashes? Have you ever had enlarged lymph nodes? Have you had symptoms or diseases related to the eyes, ears, nose, mouth, or throat?

Sometimes wheezing can be a symptom of congestive heart failure. Have you had any heart symptoms, such as chest pain, palpitations, or swelling in the feet? Do you develop shortness of breath in the middle of the night? Do you require two pillows to sleep comfortably? Have you had rheumatic fever, a heart attack, a heart-valve abnormality, a heart murmur, an irregular heart rate, or heart failure?

Have you had any stomach or abdominal symptoms, such as heartburn, nausea, vomiting, stomach pain, diarrhea, or constipation? Heartburn and reflux symptoms can be related to asthma exacerbations. Have you ever had kidney stones, arthritic symptoms, or neurological symptoms?

Questions about occupational and environmental exposures will be asked next because certain types of exposures can cause asthma. The questions begin with the year you were born and your place of birth. The questions also include your past summer jobs, military service, and first job. The questions will continue with a review of your chronological list of jobs. Specific questions will be asked about exposure to hazardous dusts and to chemicals or toxic fumes, vapors or mists. If you had an exposure, how much was the exposure? When did it occur? What about your office environment? If you were exposed, when was the exposure in relation to the onset of the asthma symptoms? What was the level of exposure on a scale of low to high, and what was the duration of exposure?

What are your hobbies? These may be causes of asthma. Sometimes it's helpful to know what type of work your spouse or other members of your household are doing.

The final portion of the inquiry focuses on the medications that you might be taking. It's helpful to know the name of each medication, the dose, when it was started, and the reason for taking it. Several medications can cause wheezing, cough, or even an asthma attack.

———

Fred was in his 70s, and was fit and healthy. One afternoon he developed wheezing. It stopped after a few minutes, and he ignored it.

But he kept having repeated episodes and it was getting worse. Over the next few days, an episode of wheezing that wouldn't stop landed him in the emergency room.

"What's going on?" Fred said with a gasp as he tried to catch his breath.

"Do you have asthma?" the ER doctor asked.

"No, I've never been sick, and I don't even take any pills."

The wheezing worsened, and he was admitted to the hospital for observation. He was treated with a hand-held nebulizer and intravenous fluids. During the next 24 hours, the wheezing resolved.

The doctor began asking questions. "You said you never had asthma. Are you allergic to any foods, medications or pollen?"

"I used to have itchy eyes during the fall pollen season," Fred said. "My daughter is allergic to spring pollens. I've never been allergic to any medicines or foods."

"Have you ever developed wheezing with cold weather or with exercise?"

"No."

"What about work? Did you ever develop wheezing from something at work?" the doctor asked.

"I'm retired now. I was a supervisor at a chemical plant for 40 years, and never had any problem with the dusts or fumes."

"No clues yet," the doctor said. "I don't think it's a tumor because it happened too quickly without any other symptoms. Have you gone to the doctor during the past few weeks?"

"I went to the eye doctor for a check-up."

"What did the doctor find?"

"Nothing much. I had some mild glaucoma." Fred said.

"That could be important. Did you get some eye drops?"

"Yes, I had been using them for a few days before the wheezing started," Fred said. "What does that have to do with anything?"

"Glaucoma is increased pressure in the eye," the doctor explained. "Some types of eye drops called beta-blockers are used to decrease the pressure. These beta-blockers are also commonly used to decrease blood pressure and slow the heart rate."

"I don't have high blood pressure, and I don't take pills," Fred said.

"Yes, but these beta-blockers have the opposite effect on the airways; they constrict them, causing bronchospasm and wheezing."

"Amazing!" Fred exclaimed.

"You mean the eye drops I was using went into the blood stream, and then into the airways and constricted them?" Fred asked. "Not only that, they were powerful enough to send me to the hospital?"

"Yup, that's it."

Fred was given another type of eye drops that controlled his glaucoma. His wheezing episodes did not recur.

Be sure to tell your doctor about all types of medications, because some of them can have unusual side effects. In addition, be sure to mention vitamins and supplements that you take because you may be a person who is sensitive to their effects, and some of them can be toxic in high doses.

At this point, you have answered the questions; it's helpful to summarize the story of your illness and add any additional information that might help establish a diagnosis.

The second component of the diagnostic process is the physical examination. Your doctor will take your vital signs – blood pressure, pulse, temperature, respiratory rate, and oxygen-saturation value. Respiratory rate is often increased in asthma. The oxygen- saturation test measures the percentage of oxygen contained in the blood hemoglobin. Values over 95% are normal, and values of less than 85% are considered much below normal. With mild-to-moderate asthma, the oxygen saturation is often normal; however, a decrease in oxygen saturation in someone with asthma signals a severe attack because the constricted airways are not allowing a sufficient amount of air into the lungs.

Your fingernails will be examined for a bluish color, which may mean low oxygen. Your ears, eyes, and throat will be examined for any abnormalities. Your neck and tops of your shoulders will be palpated to determine if any lymph nodes are enlarged.

The stethoscope is used to detect abnormal sounds. With asthma, there will be wheezes during an expiratory breath. If there are wheezes during an inspiratory breath, it's a sign of more severe asthma, as the constriction of the airways becomes more widespread. Crackling sounds will not be heard unless there is pneumonia.

For asthma, the rest of the physical examination is usually normal, although your heart will be examined and your feet inspected for swelling.

––––

The third component of the diagnostic process is a series of sequential tests to determine the specific type of asthma you may have.

Laboratory studies include a complete blood cell count that is used to search for eosinophils, which are white blood cells that contain red granules and often represent an allergic component to the asthma. The total white blood cell count may be increased during an infection or if someone is taking a corticosteroid medicine such as prednisone. A corticosteroid inhaler given at recommended dose will not increase the total white blood cell count. Tests that measure liver and kidney function are usually normal.

With asthma, the chest x-rays are often normal, but they do help determine whether pneumonia is present. If the chest x-ray is abnormal, you would probably undergo a high-resolution chest CT scan to further characterize the abnormality. If the small bronchioles are thought to be causing the airflow obstruction, the CT scan will be obtained during inspiration and expiration to determine whether there is trapped air in the lung from narrow or obliterated small bronchiole airways.

The diagnostic process also consists of pulmonary function tests, or PFTs. The forced vital capacity, or FVC, measures the amount of air in the lungs. This test is usually normal with mild or moderate asthma because most people with asthma can breathe in enough air – the problem is people are unable to breathe out enough air because of the constricted and bronchospastic airways. This test will be decreased in severe asthma.

The forced expired volume in one second, or FEV_1, measures the amount of air expired in one second. This is the single best test for asthma because it measures the amount of air that can be blown out with each breath and measures the degree of airway obstruction. It's like blowing out a candle, except the FEV_1 test yields useful numbers.

For an asthma evaluation, this test is repeated after you breathe in a bronchodilator medicine from a hand-held nebulizer or an inhaler. This test is called a post-bronchodilator FEV_1, and if it shows an increase of 12% or more than the original FEV_1, it can confirm reactive airways or asthma.

Peak flow is another common test for asthma. It's just what it sounds like – the highest flow of air that you can blow out as fast as you can. It's easy to measure with a hand-held device, so it's a popular test used at home to monitor asthma.

The baseline lung volume test may be helpful for asthma. With this test, you quietly breathe into a tube attached to the pulmonary function machine and intermittently take deep breaths blowing out your air. This test can also be done in a plethysmography chamber, or body box, where you sit inside a clear-walled chamber and breathe quickly, like panting, into a tube. The total lung capacity is the vital capacity plus the air that is left in your lungs, and is usually normal for asthma, except when it's severe. The residual volume is an important test for asthma because it measures how much air is left in your lungs after you blow out as much as you can. This amount of air is increased in asthma because it's trapped behind the constricted airways and remains in the lungs.

The final pulmonary function test is the diffusing capacity, which measures the ability of the lungs to exchange oxygen from the air into the blood circulating in the lungs. This test is usually normal in asthma, or may be increased because of increased blood flow into the upper lung regions.

These pulmonary function tests are designated as "percent predicted," which means your tests are compared to hundreds of individuals who do not have lung disease. Values of 80% predicted or above are normal. Mild decrease is from 60% to 80% predicted; moderate decrease is from 50% to 79% predicted for the vital capacity and 40% to 79% for the diffusing capacity. Values less than 40% predicted are considered to show severe lung impairment.

The diagnosis of asthma can often be established by reviewing the symptoms, the wheezing heard through the stethoscope, and the pulmonary function tests. Sometimes special tests are needed to confirm the specific type of asthma.

One of these is called allergy testing, which can be performed with a series of skin tests or blood tests for specific immune globulins. These tests may show more positive results than a person is aware of, but they will provide a good baseline to avoid or keep these types of exposures to a minimum.

Another specialized test is called an inhalation challenge test. Methacholine is given through a nebulizer at a small dose to determine whether there is a decrease in the one-second expired test, or FEV_1, and the dose is gradually increased. Methacholine has the opposite reaction from the bronchodilator medication, and instead of opening the airways, it causes constriction of the airways in people with asthma. The dose is increased three times or it's stopped if there is a 20% decrease in the FEV_1 test. This test will confirm the diagnosis of asthma, and is used for people who have suspected symptoms but who have normal pulmonary function tests. The test is negative if there is no change in the FEV_1 from the beginning of the test to the end.

Another challenge test is to utilize a specific amount of exercise on a treadmill or bicycle. The FEV_1 is measured before and after the exercise. A 20% decrease constitutes a positive test for hyper-reactive airways and asthma. This test can also be performed with cold air.

Inhalation challenge tests can also be used to confirm a diagnosis of occupational asthma. Although this test is not common and is performed only in specialized academic settings, it involves using the suspected inciting agent such as a chemical from the workplace or dust from cedar shingles.

———

Carl Upton was a hard worker. He had been working in factories for years and never had any lung problem; however, one day he went to see Dr. Jeeves because he had been wheezing at night.

"You might have asthma or heart failure," the doctor said. "When did the wheezing begin?"

"I've noticed it during the past few days," Carl replied. "I've never been sick and never had asthma. No one in the family has asthma. I've never smoked cigarettes. My heart's good."

"Your lungs sound normal today," Dr. Jeeves said. "Your heart sounds normal and your heart tests are normal. Your pulmonary function tests are normal, and your chest x-ray is normal."

"So, what's going on?" Carl asked.

"Let's monitor the situation with a peak-flow meter, and see what turns up."

Carl returned home and began charting peak flow measurements. It was easy because he just blew into a flow meter and the findings were recorded and stored on the computer. He also marked down what he was doing when he measured the peak flow.

"Let's review your printout," the Dr. Jeeves said. "Hmm, there seems to be a pattern."

"I think I see what you're saying," Carl said. "I'm normal first thing Monday morning, then the number decreases dramatically after two to three hours at work, and then goes back to normal by the afternoon. That's strange."

"But, look here," Dr. Jeeves said as he pointed to the printout that showed Carl's test results during the late-night hours. "Your peak flow decreases again very dramatically during the night."

"So, what does this mean?"

"You may have become sensitized to something at work that's causing occupational asthma."

"How could it be something at work?" Carl asked, "It's better in the afternoon and happens in the middle of the night, completely away from work."

"It's called a dual reaction and means that your airways have developed sensitivity to a specific chemical. After the immune cells in the airways become sensitized, they begin to secrete toxic substances when exposed to this chemical, and during ten hours, these toxic materials eventually cause bronchospasm and wheezing."

"OK, Doc, that's confusing, but it sounds like my lungs are sensitized to something at the work, except I'm not exposed to anything," Carl said.

"Sometimes, you may not know," Dr. Jeeves said. "Ask your industrial hygienist or your safety officer about your work. Review the material safety data sheets, or MSDS, that are available for all your workplace exposures. If you work by yourself or with two or three other workers, read the label very carefully for every word to find out about potential respiratory adverse effects. You can also search the internet for information about these exposures."

"Sounds like a lot of work, but it's probably worth my time," Carl said. "You might be right about something at work. Now that I think about it, I recently started a new project. I need to find out more about the job."

Carl had been assigned to a special furniture-finishing project in the varnishing shed. John Marsden, the safe work-practice supervisor, had been transferred to another factory and his replacement had not yet talked to Carl about his new project and the safety procedures required.

Carl went to see the new supervisor, Josh Armstrong.

"Let's review your job," Josh said. "How are you varnishing the furniture?"

"I mix Part A solution with Part B solution and quickly apply it to the furniture before it hardens," Carl said.

"Do you wear a respirator?"

"I wear one of the paper masks that I used in the past."

"Let's review that varnishing product," Josh said. "It looks like you are working with a varnish that contains TDI, which is a chemical with a long name, toluene diisocyanate. This can be a powerful asthma sensitizer, which means that people's lungs can become sensitized to TDI, and every new exposure will cause bronchospasm and wheezing. It also has the dual-response effect, which means it occurs Monday morning, disappears, and occurs again at night, and disappears by Friday."

"Whoa, that's me!" Carl exclaimed.

"Some chemicals and substances such as TDI used for polystyrene foam products and epoxy, where component A is mixed with component B, are capable of causing sensitivity," Josh said. "One or two exposures usually do not cause symptoms, but repeated exposures during weeks or months can cause sensitization. Once sensitization occurs, every time a person is exposed to that specific chemical, wheezing will occur."

"That's what happened to me," Carl said.

"We need to fix the problem now," Josh said. "You will not return to that job. We are going to change the project so that the varnishing process is performed in an enclosed area by robotic machines and the exhaust air is neutralized."

Carl returned to his previous work assignment and experienced no more wheezing episodes. The lung problem was discovered in time. He had not been exposed long enough to cause permanent lung dysfunction. His lungs and pulmonary function tests were normal.

———

All wheezes may not be asthma. Some conditions mimic asthma, and because they do, they can be difficult to diagnose. It's important to diagnose these conditions because mimics of asthma do not respond to asthma medicines. In some situations, they may require surgery, as in the event of a tumor, or they may require other medications or none at all. There's no reason to expose yourself to medicines that have no beneficial effect for you.

One of the mimics is called vocal cord dysfunction syndrome. A person with this syndrome has no structural abnormalities with the vocal cords, but they close during an inspiratory breath, causing a wheezing sound. Two symptom pattern tests can diagnose vocal cord dysfunction syndrome: one, if the wheezing sound disappears when the person is asleep; and two, if the patient wheezes during inspiration (breathing in) instead of expiration (breathing out), as occurs in typical asthma. The shape of the flow-volume loop obtained during the pulmonary function tests may be helpful as it may show flattening of the inspiratory portion of the loop. The diagnosis can be confirmed with a laryngoscope that can show closing of the vocal cords during inspiration.

Some people with vocal cord dysfunction syndrome have a history of psychological stress or trauma. Vocal cord dysfunction syndrome is seen in overstressed teenagers, especially those near competitive success, as a graceful way to exit high-pressure situations and not face failure.

People with psychological troubles sometimes complicate the diagnosis by becoming angry at their physicians for considering a psychological diagnosis, as many patients have subconsciously developed the wheezing to gain sympathetic attention from family or friends, and the stress and strong emotion may trigger real asthma in some people. These individuals, though, have normal lungs and unknown to them, have created an expiratory wheezing sound through their vocal cords that can be triggered by irritant exposures and other typical asthma triggers.

The major issue in these situations is that individuals may receive extensive, potentially dangerous treatment for asthma including intravenous corticosteroid treatment in the emergency room and sometimes ongoing for months or years. Yet that treatment is not needed. Treatment for vocal cord dysfunction syndrome should instead focus on psychiatric counseling and speech therapy.

A second mimic of asthma is the persistent cough. Although it indicates inflammation in the bronchial airways, not all coughing causes constriction of the airways and wheezing. Persistent cough that may not be asthma most often occurs in small children with recurring respiratory infections.

A third asthma mimic is chronic obstructive pulmonary disease, or COPD. Caused primarily by smoking, COPD has two main conditions: chronic bronchitis from irritated and inflamed bronchial airways, and emphysema, which is damage and coalescence of the spherical structures in the lung called alveoli. Damage to the alveoli causes airways to collapse, which can result in airflow obstruction.

The bronchitis is called chronic bronchitis because it doesn't go away, as asthma symptoms can, and is characterized by daily cough with phlegm, especially in the morning. Most people with COPD have both chronic bronchitis and emphysema, although one may be more prominent. The chronic bronchitis causes morning phlegm and wheezing, while the emphysema causes decreased to absent breath sounds. COPD is not asthma, and although the symptoms can ease or worsen on a given day, they don't go away.

Other diseases and conditions that cause narrowing of the airways and mimic asthma include inhaling foreign substances into the lungs. Another involves the very small bronchiole airways, such as those that occur after unusual viral pneumonias or toxic fume inhalation, or are associated with some of the connective tissue diseases such as rheumatoid arthritis. If you remember the story about Pete in the first chapter, unusual tumors can also sometimes cause wheezing.

If you find that you don't have asthma, but you have a mimic of asthma, the five steps can help you manage the situation successfully, just as Pete did.

———

Let's continue Billy Norton's story from Chapter 2. He had sustained a terrible asthma attack, and had returned home from the emergency room to begin learning about asthma.

He learned about the two components of airway inflammation and wheezing from bronchospasm. He then went to a lung specialist, Dr. Sarah Whitney, to find out more and undergo the diagnostic process.

"Tell me what happened when you developed the wheezing," Dr. Whitney said.

"I had some chest tightness for a couple of days, but I didn't any pay attention to it," Billy said. "Suddenly it worsened, sending me to the emergency room."

"Did you have cough and phlegm?"

"I had a cough when the wheezing started but not before. There was no phlegm."

"Did you have a fever, chills or the feeling of a respiratory infection?" Dr. Whitney asked. "This can sometimes be a trigger of asthma."

"No, nothing like that. I've never been sick, and I never had asthma."

"Anyone in your family with asthma or allergies?"

"I remember my mother used an inhaler when I was growing up, and my grandmother had asthma."

"Do you have any allergies to foods, medicines, or pollen?"

"I sometimes hear a raspy sound in my chest when I drink a cold milk shake, but it goes away in a few minutes," Billy said. "I'm not allergic to any medicines, and I'm not allergic to my dog."

"Any other allergies?" Dr. Whitney asked.

"Sometimes, when I was younger, I had episodes of sneezing about five to ten times in a row, but nothing else happened. I'm allergic to nickel because I developed red spots underneath my watch when I was a kid."

"You've probably had reactive-airway syndrome or hyperresponsive airways most of your life. This is common and occurs in about 20% of people. The airways are more sensitive than normal and react to inhaled materials more readily. People develop chest colds instead of head colds. They are also prone to skin rashes and some allergies."

"What happens to people with reactive airways?" Billy asked.

"For most people, it's an annoying problem that generally takes care of itself, causing periodic discomfort from colds and irritant exposures."

"Does it cause asthma?"

"In itself, no," Dr. Whitney said. "About eight percent of the population has asthma, and individuals with reactive airways have a higher frequency of developing asthma, but most of these individuals go through life without ever developing asthma.

Sometimes a viral or bacterial pneumonia can cause an asthma attack. So, let's get a chest x-ray to find out?"

The doctor reviewed the x-ray films with Billy. The lungs appeared normal.

"I would like to obtain some routine blood tests to find out other causes of asthma and specifically to search for an increase in a special white blood cell called an eosinophil. These cells are sometimes increased in people with allergic asthma."

When Billy's blood tests came back, he and Dr. Whitney reviewed them.

"All the blood tests look good," Dr. Whitney said. "Your liver and kidney functions are normal. Your white blood cells are normal and there is no increase in the eosinophils. We'll send you for some pulmonary function tests to see about those reactive airways."

They again reviewed the test results together.

"Your vital capacity measures the amount of air you can blow out of your lungs, and it's normal. Your FEV_1 test that measures the amount of air you can blow out in one second is decreased, so the ratio of the FEV_1 to the forced vital capacity or FEV_1/FVC is decreased."

"What does that mean?" Billy asked.

"In asthma, the airways are constricted and narrow so you can't blow out as much air as usual which means the FEV_1 test is going to be decreased," Dr. Whitney explained. "But, look what happened when you take the bronchodilator medicine that relaxes the circular muscles surrounding the airways, the FEV_1 increased by 20%. That's reactive airways."

"Does that mean I have asthma?"

"Probably, let's look at some additional tests," Dr. Whitney said. "Your total lung capacity is normal; however, the residual volume which is the amount of air left over after you blow out is increased, which means that some of the air is trapped behind the constricted airways."

"That makes sense," Billy said.

"What about this diffusion test? It's actually above normal."

"That's the diffusing capacity, which measures the ability of your red blood cells to take up oxygen. In asthma, this test is usually normal and may be above normal because the upper lungs become involved in oxygen exchange."

"So, what's next?" Billy asked.

"You probably have typical adult-onset asthma. You don't need other diagnostic tests now. We can obtain allergy testing and other specific tests if needed in the future."

"How do I treat it?" Billy asked anxiously as he waited for some good news.

———

Billy had gone through the diagnostic process and had understood the testing and the reasons for all of the testing. We'll find out about his treatment management plan in the next chapter.

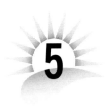

Treatment Options for Mild, Moderate or Severe Asthma:
Rescue and Maintenance

The good news is that asthma is treatable and you can manage it. If that doesn't sound right to you, you might be remembering a time, as short a time ago as the 1980s, when people considered asthma a disease that would limit people. Specialists now say that, with treatment, 95 percent of people with asthma, all but those with the most severe cases, can do pretty much anything.

The breakthrough occurred in 1989 when the National Asthma Education and Prevention Program, or NAEPP, was created through the National Institutes of Health. The program was formed to address what was regarded as an asthma epidemic. The NAEPP issued guidelines that advised physicians to treat asthma not just as bronchospasm, but as an underlying airway inflammatory condition. The program continues to provide updated information about asthma. Since the NAEPP started issuing guidelines on treatment and reviewed them, the mortality rate among asthma patients has decreased.

Treating asthma as an underlying inflammatory condition means that treatment for most asthma involves not only a bronchodilator, but also an inhaled corticosteroid. You cannot, however, interchange and substitute these medicines. You will need both.

You use the bronchodilator to rescue you from an asthma attack. It works quickly to relax the smooth muscles around the bronchi when they go into bronchospasm. You use the corticosteroid inhaler to reduce the underlying airway inflammation and the chronic vulnerability to bronchospasm. Inhaled corticosteroids maintain your underlying bronchial health, and regular use will help you manage your asthma.

The corticosteroids used for asthma are anti-inflammatory steroids. They are not anabolic steroids, which have a bad reputation because athletes may abuse them to bulk-up muscle. Inhaled corticosteroids for asthma are considered safe. They do not circulate widely through the blood, but are deposited on the bronchial airways and stay there decreasing the amount of inflammation. After 40 to 50 years of experience with these medications, there is no long-term evidence for atrophy or thinning of the bronchial airways. They are also now considered first-line therapy for children.

Inhaled corticosteroids deliver a much smaller dose than pills. The inhaler dose is usually about one microgram, which is one millionth of a gram, while the prednisone dose is given in multiple milligrams, and one milligram is one thousandth of a gram. It's important to remember that the corticosteroid inhaler takes several days to take effect and it must be used daily to be effective.

Inhaled corticosteroids are, however, a big improvement over the past maintenance treatment available, which was called theophylline. Some patients whose asthma is stable and are taking theophylline have continued it, but since it requires regular blood tests to monitor its action and has many interactions with other drugs, it has not been used much over the last decade.

The use of these two classes of medication, bronchodilators and inhaled corticosteroids, is determined by the type and severity of the asthma. The definitions of asthma that are generally used include mild intermittent, mild persistent, moderate persistent, and severe persistent. We'll go through typical treatments for each category.

Mild Intermittent Asthma

Jill Anderson developed mild intermittent asthma. Let's examine how she approached her diagnosis and treatment.

———

Jill experienced occasional tightness in her chest and wheezing. She was talking to her family doctor.

"How long have you had these symptoms?" Dr. Whitmore asked.

"I've noticed them during the past two to three years when I develop a cold," Jill answered.

"Do you have shortness of breath or a cough with phlegm?"

"No, and I have no other symptoms."

"You may have asthma," the doctor said.

Tests confirmed she had mild asthma. Her chest x-ray and pulmonary function tests were normal, but her one-second expired volume, or FEV_1, increased after she used the bronchodilator medicine.

"What are the treatment options?" Jill asked.

"Let's talk about them," Dr. Whitmore said. "First, it appears to be typical adult asthma with no allergic triggers. The natural course of this type of asthma is generally fairly benign, with intermittent attacks triggered by respiratory infections and irritant smoke or fumes. One option is no treatment. However, since these symptoms are uncomfortable and can be treated successfully, I would suggest the second option of using an inhaler when you develop the wheezing."

"What's in the inhaler?" Jill asked.

"It's a bronchodilator," the doctor explained, "which is a long word for a medicine that relaxes the circular smooth muscles surrounding each airway so they open and you can blow out the air from your lungs. The medicine is put into an inhaler or can be mixed with saline and added to a hand-held nebulizer. An inhaler would be best for you."

"How effective is it?"

"You have to learn to use it correctly," Dr. Whitmore emphasized. "You first blow out your air, then open your mouth and squeeze the inhaler deeply, breathing in the puff of medicine. It sounds simple, but sometimes people blow out instead of breathing in, and the medicine goes into the air or into the mouth, which doesn't change the narrowed airways."

"That's helpful to know."

"Two puffs are usually recommended. If used properly, the medicine begins to improve the wheezing within one to three minutes and lasts for several hours. For mild intermittent asthma, an inhaler is usually all that's needed, and can be used two or three times a day when the wheezing occurs and stopped after the wheezing stops."

"Are there other treatment options?" Jill asked.

"Corticosteroid medicines are powerful anti-inflammatory medicines that can be very helpful for more advanced asthma," Dr. Whitmore said. "For you, I would recommend using the bronchodilator inhaler because it's easy to use, it's safe, and you only have symptoms two or three times a year."

"What are the risks of the bronchodilator inhaler?" Jill asked.

"If you only use the inhaler when you have wheezing, and no more than three or four times per day for a few days, the risk is very low," the doctor said. "It relaxes the airways' circular smooth muscles, but it has the opposite effect on the smooth muscle of the heart and can speed it up, especially if too much is used. In the past, the inhalers had a large heart component. The newer inhalers have more of the dilator component and less of the heart component. So, you may not have any effect, or you may have mild speeding of the heart or jittery hands for a few minutes."

"I didn't notice anything when I did the pulmonary function test, so I don't think I'll have any problem," Jill said.

"People may be allergic to the sulfate preservative in the inhaler, and the wheezing may worsen, but this is rare," Dr. Whitmore added.

"I don't have a sulfate allergy, so I'm going to use the inhaler when I need it for episodes of wheezing," Jill concluded.

———

Jill did a great job asking questions about what medicine to use, how it works, when to use it, and how much to use.

Sue, as you recall from Chapter 1, had exercised-induced asthma. Since exercise was the only asthma trigger, her treatment would be similar to Jill's. She uses her bronchodilator before exercise. Sue also uses a slow, gradual seven-minute warm-up before exercising or competing in an athletic event.

It appears that the bronchial airway cells that cause exercise-induced asthma can be blunted if people use several minutes of slow warm-up, just enough to dampen the release of the asthma-producing substances from mast cells, but not too much to cause bronchospasm and wheezing. After this type of warm-up, most people can exercise as vigorously as they wish.

Mild Persistent Asthma

Jill didn't experience tightness in her chest or wheezing very often, mostly after colds, so her asthma was intermittent. People have mild persistent asthma when their asthma attacks are mild but occur on a weekly, or more frequent basis; for example, if they need to use their inhaler more than two times a week, or they wake up more than twice a month coughing and feeling chest tightness. The line between intermittent and persistent is a judgment call between you and your doctor.

As we learned with Jill's experience, a bronchodilator inhaler may be sufficient for someone who has intermittent asthma because it takes care of the immediate wheezing and tightness. But when asthma attacks occur more frequently, a person should also start taking an anti-inflammatory steroid inhaler, which will reduce the underlying vulnerability of the bronchial airways to bronchospasm.

As mentioned previously, you need to take this inhaled corticosteroid daily to be effective. Think of it as the breathing equivalent to brushing your teeth.

Follow directions when you take your medications. For most inhaled corticosteroids, you can use a spacer and rinse out your mouth with water afterward to prevent one common side-effect – a yeast infection called thrush. A spacer holds the inhaler medicine in a large-diameter tubular device. You then breathe in the medicine contained in the spacer, which can improve the amount of medicine delivered to the airways.

Remember not to swallow the water you use to rinse your mouth. Some of the inhaled corticosteroid can settle on your vocal cords and cause intermittent hoarseness. If that happens, you should talk to your doctor about changing the type of steroid you take because there are several choices.

Inhaled steroids come in three forms: puffers, which deliver a metered dose, dry- powder inhalers, and liquid formulas for nebulizers.

QVAR® (beclomethasone), Alvesco® (ciclesonide), and Flovent® (fluticasone propionate) are examples of puffers. Pulmicort® (budesonide) and Asmanex® (mometasone) are examples of powders. Pulmicort® also comes in liquid form for nebulizers. Other inhaled steroid formulas were used, but they were discontinued because they contained chlorofluorocarbons, or CFCs, which harmed the ozone layer in the atmosphere.

Pulmicort® is one of the steroid inhalers for pregnant women. As mentioned before, pregnancy can affect a woman's asthma. This medication, like other inhaled steroids, has differing dose strengths that can be used to meet asthma severity.

You and your doctor will be able to determine what dosage level you need, and be sure to review the specific way to take the medicine, and know what it can and cannot do. Remember, an inhaled corticosteroid will not help you during an actual asthma attack. You need your rescue bronchodilator for that.

Parents of children with asthma often worry that their child will not grow as tall if they take an inhaled corticosteroid. A large study showed that during the first year of taking an inhaled steroid, children did not grow as much as they might be expected to by one centimeter less, as projected by growth chart curves. They did, however, seem to make it up later as their bodies adjusted to the medication.

A new class of drugs, called leukotriene blockers, provides another option for some children with mild persistent asthma. Many parents want to try leukotriene blockers first because they're worried about their child's growth.

Singulair® (montelukast) is one of these leukotriene blockers. When external allergens such as pollens are inhaled by someone with allergic asthma, a toxic substance in the form of leukotriene is released that causes inflammation and bronchospasm. So, medicines that block the leukotriene release will prevent the inflammation and bronchospasm. Although the leukotriene pathway appears to be a potent signal for asthma, on average, leukotriene blockers do not work as well as steroids.

For children, Singulair® comes as chew tablets and as sprinkles that parents can add to food for children as young as one year. Children who take this medication should be watched for changes in mood, as the FDA has reported some relationship between this medication and depression.

Moderate Persistent Asthma

Someone with moderate persistent asthma needs to use the rescue bronchodilator inhaler every day or has uncontrolled asthma after using inhaled steroids.

For these people, there are additional treatment options. One came available about ten years ago when a pharmaceutical company changed the molecule of the most common bronchodilator so that it worked for

12 hours, not the standard four to six. These long-acting beta-agonists (LABAs) changed people's lives because instead of needing many puffs from an inhaler every day, and waking up at night coughing and feeling tight in the chest, a person could take one puff and sleep through the night. Examples of these long-acting bronchodilators are Serevent® (salmeterol) and Foradil® (formoterol).

These long-acting bronchodilators have met with some controversy, however, as a study found that people who take them had a higher incidence of deaths and near deaths from asthma attacks. Since then, all the long-acting bronchodilator medicines are now required to have a "black-box" warning label about this increased risk. The big question then remained, would a combined inhaled corticosteroid along with a long-acting bronchodilator decrease the risk?

These combination drugs do now exist. There are three: Advair® (fluticasone and salmeterol), Symbicort® (budesonide and formoterol), and Dulera® (mometasone and formoterol). They can be obtained in different strengths. Advair®, for example, has four dosage levels.

Most people feel comfortable about these "combination" drugs. There has been an increase in their use and a decrease in deaths from asthma; however, these combination inhalers still carry the "black-box" warning because of the long-acting bronchodilator.

Treatment guidelines for teenagers include a recommendation for the combined inhaler so they will not have to remember to take two inhalers. These types of inhalers also appear to work best for people with severe asthma.

Severe Persistent Asthma

In some situations, people may have severe persistent asthma, which is defined as nighttime awakenings with asthma symptoms almost every night, limited daily activities because of the asthma, and asthma flare-ups that require use of oral steroids two or more times a year. There are additional options for treatment of severe persistent asthma.

The first option is best for allergic asthma, in which allergens trigger asthma. The drug is Xolair® (omalizumab), and it removes specific immunoglobulin E (IgE) proteins from the blood. IgE proteins signal the mast cells, which are immune cells in the bronchial airways, that an allergen is present. The mast cells respond with a toxic allergic reaction – inflammation and bronchospasm. The Xolair® medication detects the circulating IgE in the blood and binds to it where the IgE would bind to the mast cell. So, it's neutralized and the Xolair®-IgE complex is eliminated.

Xolair® has been shown to decrease asthma attacks. It's an individualized treatment. It's effective for some individuals with asthma, while others may not show improvement. It's a solution that is injected and is given every two to four weeks. Before embarking on this therapy, a person needs to be tested for specific circulating IgE in the blood. If there is no excessive IgE, the medicine will not be effective and is not recommended.

The traditional immunotherapy with the standard allergy shots is another allergy-specific treatment. Once the allergy has been identified, a person is given an injection of a tiny amount of the allergen, which is gradually increased over time until there is no longer an asthma response to the allergen.

Although this therapy works well for people with itchy eyes and watery nose from hay fever or for people who develop anaphylactic shock from bee stings, the therapy is controversial for asthma. It may not be effective because there appears to be a difference in allergic pathways in the nose and eyes compared to the allergic pathway in the bronchial airways.

A new therapy, just approved by the FDA, called bronchial thermoplasty is for people with severe persistent asthma who have not responded to anything else. In this therapy, thermal energy is delivered through a bronchoscope to the bronchial airways to decrease the excess circular smooth muscle that is causing the airway constriction and wheezing. Three treatments are administered, each three weeks apart. This is a bronchoscopy procedure, so the treatment is performed in a bronchoscopy suite or unit and has the risks associated with bronchoscopy that include bleeding and infection, but it seems to reduce asthma attacks while keeping lung function steady.

Prednisone is the treatment of last resort for severe asthma that does not respond to anything else. We'll address prednisone in the next chapter.

Treating the Severe Asthma Attack

When a severe attack occurs, sometimes the only solution is to go to an emergency room. At the hospital, you will be treated with a nebulized albuterol bronchodilator and intravenous (IV) prednisone.

One benefit of learning how to manage your asthma through the five steps in this book is that you can learn to manage your asthma attacks at home or while traveling. Develop a plan with your doctor or asthma nurse specialist to treat asthma attacks outside the ER as part of your overall asthma action plan. You want to keep out of the ER if you can. Develop a color-coded plan to make it easy and workable.

If you feel an attack coming on and want to try treating it at home first, start by taking a few extra puffs of your bronchodilator and holding your breath a few seconds more than usual. It's the same medication that you would receive at the hospital. You might try a home hand-held nebulizer for this purpose. If you have pills of prednisone, follow the directions on your plan list as you developed with your doctor or asthma nurse as to how many you can take. Prednisone pills work just as well as the intravenous form. Then, continue to use the bronchodilator until the prednisone decreases the inflammation and improves your breathing.

With planning and confidence in yourself, you can prevent your fear of an asthma attack and avoid allowing asthma to limit your activities and travel. The good news about asthma is that it's treatable for the vast majority of people.

The ER is always there for your backup.

———

Let's continue with Billy's story.

He had completed his diagnostic evaluation, as we discussed in the last chapter. He made an appointment to see his doctor for ongoing treatment, but suddenly developed a high fever, severe cough with green sputum, and wheezing so bad that he had to go to the ER.

"We have a severe asthma attack and an emergency!" the triage nurse exclaimed. "Send Billy to the crash cart room and call anesthesia."

Billy's airways were so constricted that he couldn't breathe in any air. His oxygen level had plummeted and his carbon dioxide level had risen to dangerous levels. It was too late to wait for the medicines to take effect. He had to have a tube inserted into his trachea and placed on assisted ventilation, which meant he was hooked up to a machine to deliver oxygen and eliminate the carbon dioxide. The pressure required to deliver oxygen into his lungs was so high that he had to have paralytic medicines to loosen his muscles. But, within a few minutes, the emergency was over and the ventilation machine had taken over.

The portable chest x-ray showed pneumonia in both lungs. Blood samples were drawn to discover the type of bacteria causing the pneumonia and two types of intravenous antibiotics were started. At the same time, he needed treatment for the asthma.

"Have the respiratory therapist use a bronchodilator aerosol through the ventilator, and have them do chest physical therapy to assure the airway secretions are cleared," the ER doctor told the nursing staff. "Add the corticosteroid to the bag of intravenous fluid."

The intravenous medications began to take effect, and the antibiotics would stop the toxic bacteria from causing further damage. Over time, the paralyzing medicines were discontinued, and the inspired oxygen level was decreased from 100% to 40%. After 12 hours, the tube was pulled out of Billy's trachea and he was taken off the ventilator, as he was able to maintain a good oxygen level and normal carbon dioxide level on his own.

The steroid medicine was changed from the intravenous form to prednisone at 40 mg each day on a decreasing tapering dose schedule. After several days, Billy was discharged. He continued to take the antibiotic for a complete ten-day course. He then returned to see Dr. Whitney.

"I don't remember much, but I think I had a serious asthma attack," Billy said.

"Yes, it's just as well you don't remember, but the pneumonia really triggered your airways and clamped them shut. You were successfully treated, and the pneumonia is resolving," Dr. Whitney reassured him.

You have typical adult asthma that may occur from respiratory infections, as you found out last week. It may also occur without an obvious trigger or from irritant chemical exposures. You don't have a postnasal drip or gastroesophageal reflux that could trigger the asthma."

"Where do we do from here?" Billy asked.

"We need to review using the anti-inflammatory inhaler that was started while you were in the hospital," the doctor said. "The bronchodilator inhaler is useful for mild wheezing that may occur occasionally, but this new inhaler will prevent you from having so many attacks."

"What's it called?"

"It's a corticosteroid, or steroid, inhaler," Dr. Whitney said. "In the past, we only had tablets of steroid medicine and they could cause serious side effects. Now we have it in inhaled form, and when used at recommended doses, it doesn't enter the blood stream to cause the adverse effects."

"That sounds like a real breakthrough," Billy commented.

"Yes, it's been the biggest advancement in asthma treatment in decades," the doctor said. "Keep in mind, though, that just because it comes in an inhaler doesn't mean it's the same as your bronchodilator inhaler. It's almost opposite. It has no short-term effect and does not open up the airways after a few minutes, but it has a powerful, long-term, anti-inflammation effect that begins after a few days, with maximal benefit in two weeks."

"What do you mean?" Billy asked.

"It's a preventive medicine. The aerosol is deposited on the inflamed airways that are causing the asthma, and over time, neutralizes the inflammation, stopping the wheezing. Therefore, it must be used every day without interruption so that it can keep the inflammatory-producing cells in check and keep the airways from becoming inflamed."

"That makes sense," Billy said. "So, the bronchodilator inhaler opens up the airways in a few minutes, and the steroid inhaler stops the inflammation to prevent the bronchospasm and wheezing."

"Very good Billy. You should do well on your law exam."

———

Billy had successfully learned about his treatment options. After a discussion about prednisone in the next chapter, we'll find out how he monitored his asthma.

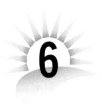

Prednisone: It Can Save Lives
Know the Benefits
and Adverse Effects

People take prednisone for a variety of disorders, and sometimes people with asthma must take this medication, so a separate section is needed to discuss the benefits and the side effects.

The adverse effects of prednisone are legendary. Most are reversible, but some are not. Some people experience no side effects. The type and severity of the adverse reactions depend on the amount of prednisone and duration of the treatment. A short course of high-dose prednisone for several days usually causes no side effects, while a long course for months or years of small- to moderate-dose prednisone is often associated with adverse effects.

Background information about corticosteroid medication is helpful to understand this powerful anti-inflammation medication. The term "cortico" is derived from the cortex of the two adrenal glands on top of the kidneys. The adrenal glands produce androgen and glucocorticoids. Both of these substances are needed for good health. Androgen is also called an anabolic steroid because it increases cell protein synthesis that increases muscle mass.

Glucocorticoids are often referred to as corticosteroids or cortisone, and they regulate cell metabolism. These corticosteroids affect the immune system by activating anti-inflammatory cell proteins, and they inhibit inflammatory cell proteins. This anti-inflammatory action is the benefit, but over time, this immune-suppression property can lead to atypical infections.

Anabolic steroids and cortisone are naturally occurring substances that are manufactured synthetically and used as medications. Anabolic steroids are used to improve muscle-mass loss in individuals with cancer or muscle-loss disorders; however, these are also the synthetic steroids used by bodybuilders and illicitly by athletes.

Cortisone is applied topically for inflamed skin; taken in tablet form for inflamed lungs, joints, and other organ systems; and used as an inhaled agent to treat asthma. In addition, there are diseases, such as Addison's, that result in loss of naturally occurring corticosteroids, so cortisone in the form of prednisone is used as a replacement.

The adrenal glands produce an equivalent of 7.5 mg of prednisone every day, which explains why doses less than 7.5 mg are less harmful. This is because the adrenal glands stop making prednisone when an external source becomes available. For example, the adrenal glands will produce 5.0 mg daily if an individual is taking 2.5 mg daily. If a person takes more than 7.5 mg of prednisone for several months or years, the adrenal glands will stop working. So, if the prednisone is stopped immediately, no corticosteroids will be available for healthy, functioning cells and the cardiovascular system will fail, causing dizziness, fainting, and a coma, if severe enough. This is the reason that the long-term prednisone dose is tapered, or decreased, slowly over time.

An increased appetite is the first effect of prednisone, as this medication goes directly to the eating center of the brain, resulting in constant signals to eat even after a meal has been eaten.

People say: "I am always hungry. I could eat anything."

This effect can be managed by maintaining a regular schedule of eating small portions. It's hard to do, but it can be helpful. Over time, the feeling of always being hungry will dissipate.

Weight gain is the second effect, which is related to the first effect as an increase in eating is going to cause weight gain, often 20 pounds, but weight gains of 40 and even 60 pounds have been reported. This weight gain can be managed with the control of the overwhelming desire to eat, which can be bypassed by staying to a regular schedule of eating small portions.

Not everyone gains weight.

———

Paul was taking high doses of prednisone, from 60 mg to 80 mg every day for a long time to treat an inflammatory lung disease. At the onset, he was determined not to gain weight or develop the typical prednisone "moon face."

Paul was intensely regimented. He didn't increase his food intake and eliminated sodium (salt) from his diet. It worked. He didn't gain a pound, and his doctor said, "You're the first person in a long time I've seen that hasn't gained weight." As Paul's story shows, use the power of your mind.

———

As weight is gained, a so-called "moon face" may develop, which is a direct effect of prednisone. This is also called a "cushingoid" appearance. The term is a reference to Cushing's syndrome, named after Dr. Harvey Cushing, who described a benign, but growing tumor in the pituitary gland that caused release of adrenal corticotrophin hormone, or ACTH, which increases adrenal gland production of cortisone.

In some people, steroid "fat pads" develop, which result from fatty-tissue buildup on the chest below the chin and below the back of the neck. The fat pad in the back is sometimes referred to by the unflattering term "buffalo hump." These effects subside as the prednisone dosage is decreased.

Other effects are purplish-red blotches and bruises that may appear on the skin of the hands and arms. These are due to fragile capillaries, as prednisone may weaken the capillary walls, causing blood to leak into the skin. They may appear spontaneously, but are generally the result of bumping into something such as a door or table. They are not harmful, but are unsightly for a few days. In some people, facial acne may develop. Both of these effects will disappear as the dosage is decreased.

Calcium loss in the bones will cause osteoporosis that can be countered by calcium, one of the biphosphonates, and an exercise program. Bone-density studies should be used for early detection of osteoporosis because, if it's severe, spinal vertebral bodies may collapse, causing pain, and this can make a person shorter.

Diabetes may occur in individuals with borderline diabetes and can be treated with anti-diabetic medications or increased insulin for diabetics. This effect is usually reversible after the prednisone is stopped, but may persist in unusual situations.

Hypertension may also occur in individuals with borderline hypertension. This is managed by anti-hypertensive medications and usually returns to baseline values after prednisone is stopped. Prednisone may cause fluid retention in the lower extremities that can be monitored, or if necessary, treated with a diuretic. Reduced sodium intake is an important part of successfully managing this effect.

During the early part of treatment, prednisone often causes the feeling of euphoria and high energy. This hyperactivity often results in the need for less sleep. These symptoms are generally transient; however, if they're persistent and cause interference with daily activities, the prednisone dose may need to be decreased.

Psychological effects such as depression or the feeling of being "out of it" or "off the wall" can be disruptive, and rather than treat these side effects with more medication, the prednisone dosage may have to be decreased. These psychological effects can be reversed as the dosage is lessened or stopped.

———

Paul, who gained no weight when he took the prednisone did, however, experience psychological effects. Every day at 4 p.m., he kiddingly told his wife not to talk to him for an hour because he was in a "bad mood." The effect gradually subsided over several days. Paul had recognized it early, anticipated it, and managed it successfully.

———

People who take prednisone for long periods are at risk of developing bacterial or fungal infections. Prednisone alters the immune system by blunting the cellular defense system that fights infections. These are often unusual and rare infections from bacteria that form branching filaments such as *Nocardia* or from fungal infections such as *Aspergillus*.

Individuals who take prednisone long term may develop *Pneumocystis*, which is a tiny parasitic organism that can massively invade the lungs. That's why, Bactrim®, a sulfa-based antibiotic, may be given three times a week to prevent this.

People who have had a past tuberculous infection and a positive tuberculin test are at risk of developing active tuberculosis. So, isoniazid, or INH, tablets may be given in conjunction with the prednisone to prevent the tuberculosis from being activated.

Another possible side effect is proximal muscle weakness which means the strong, upper-leg muscles become weak. This effect resolves as the dosage is decreased.

Two potential effects, cataracts and aseptic necrosis of the hip, are not reversible. Cataracts may occur in individuals who take prednisone long term, and surgery may be required. The reason that prednisone causes cataracts is not known.

Aseptic necrosis of the hip is associated with prednisone therapy. The term aseptic means the cause is not from an infection, and necrosis means cell death, so aseptic necrosis of the hip means the cells in the center of the ball of the hip die, and the bone becomes fragile. The exact cause is not known, although prednisone may result in expansion of the hip tissue, cutting off the circulation and leaving the internal bone cells without oxygen and nutrients. Most individuals who develop aseptic necrosis of the hip require hip replacement surgery. Maintaining a healthy weight and exercise may decrease the risk of the adverse effect.

It's important to have the complete list of side effects available because the doctor and pharmacist will not be able to list all of them during your discussion, and what they tell you may not include the one that applies to you.

You need to know what to expect when the long-term prednisone is decreased, especially if you've been taking prednisone for a year or more.

Unusual symptoms and sensations may occur that include muscle aches, fatigue, transient depression, and weakness. Usually these symptoms subside two to five days after the dose is decreased. If necessary, these symptoms can be managed by decreasing the dose from 5 mg at a time to 2.5 mg, or tapering the dose to an every-other-day schedule. An exercise program can be helpful in decreasing the impact of these withdrawal symptoms.

Prednisone is given at the lowest dose that is effective for the shortest length of time as possible to lessen the occurrence of side effects.

———

Eva Stone had asthma all of her life that she had managed successfully with her steroid inhaler and occasional use of the bronchodilator inhaler. But recently, because of the frequency and severity of her asthma attacks, she had to take prednisone tablets for several months until her asthma was once again stabilized.

"Have you had any asthma attacks recently?" Dr. Evans asked Eva during one of her follow-up visits.

"Yes, I had two or three episodes last week," Eva said. "They're not worse, but they seem to be continuing."

"Sounds like we'll have to continue your daily prednisone for now."

Eva returned the next month and reported that she still had some episodes of asthma, but not worse.

"Your weight's up ten pounds," the nurse reported.

"I was afraid of that. I eat everything in sight," Eva replied reluctantly. My face is also round, and I have some acne."

"You're having some steroid effects," Dr. Evans said. "But these attacks are continuing, so, if possible, the prednisone should be continued for a little while longer until the attacks subside."

"I can do that."

Before her next visit, Eva paid intense attention to her ravishing appetite and ate a reasonable amount at a controlled time. She was able to control her weight and had lost a pound.

"I notice these blotches and bruises on my hands," Eva said. "They don't hurt, but they're not a pretty sight."

"The skin capillaries have become fragile and break easily if you bump into something," the nurse said. "They'll disappear in a few days."

During this visit, Eva told Dr. Evans the asthma episodes had stopped.

"That's great news. Your lung examination is normal and your pulmonary function tests are normal. Let's decrease the prednisone."

"Can I stop the prednisone today?" Eva asked.

"No, you've been taking a moderately high dose for a long time. If we stop it today, your adrenal glands won't have time to catch up," Dr. Evans said. "You could develop an adrenal gland crisis resulting in collapse of your circulatory system."

"I don't want that to happen, so I'll take your advice."

Diabetes and hypertension had occurred in her family, so Eva was concerned about developing these from prednisone. She did not add salt to any of her food and decreased her sodium intake by reading the labels about sodium in foods. Her blood pressure remained normal and she had no swelling in her feet. Her blood sugar was at the high level of normal but not severe enough to warrant treatment.

During her next visit, Eva told Dr. Evans that she was puzzled because when she climbed steps, her upper-leg muscles became so weak that she could hardly make it up two flights of stairs.

"That's proximal muscle weakness," the doctor told Eva. "It's usually not serious and will resolve as we continue to decrease the prednisone dose."

During the next several weeks, Eva's weight returned to normal. Her blood sugar and her blood pressure were normal. She no longer had a "moon face," acne, or additional skin bruising.

She was feeling great and worked out at a gym near her home. It helped her deal with the side effects of the prednisone. Her exercise also gave her energy, a good feeling, and she felt in charge of her asthma again.

When the prednisone dose was decreased to a very low dose, however, Eva became concerned because she felt so weak she could hardly do her exercises. She was tired and her muscles ached. These symptoms were bad enough, but she was also depressed. All of this happened a few days after decreasing the dose.

"What's going on?" Eva asked Dr. Evans' office in an email.

"These effects sometimes occur when the dose is decreased and are usually transient. Give it a few days. Let us know if they worsen," the office staff responded.

Eva was relieved. As she was reading the reply, she realized her symptoms had started to lessen. During the next 48 hours, they disappeared.

After a few more days, the prednisone was stopped. Her asthma attacks had stopped, and she continued her daily corticosteroid inhaler.

Eva returned to her zest-filled life, and let the asthma attacks fade from her memory.

———

Prednisone can save people's lives. Yet it's important to learn as much as possible about prednisone and its adverse effects. This information will help you monitor you situation and successfully manage the medication.

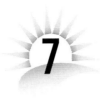

Monitor Your Asthma for Success

You have learned about asthma. You understand the diagnostic process and you know the treatment options.

Monitoring your asthma now becomes an important step for successful management so that changes can be detected and treatment can be adjusted to prevent an attack. At the same time, changes not related to asthma can be monitored to determine whether a visit to the doctor is necessary.

For people with asthma, it's important to determine which symptoms are from life's bumps and which are related to asthma. People's lives consist of intermittent aches and pains and strange feelings. You might wake up with a stuffy nose or head cold. Sleep may be disturbed by unusual pains or cramps. Sometime during the year, you might not feel quite right. You may feel run down or have mild depression. These are intermittent episodes experienced by everyone.

For asthma, wheezing is the most common symptom to monitor. It usually signals constriction of the airways. The narrowing creates the wheezing sound, meaning that it's time to use the bronchodilator inhaler. Sometimes, a cough is the first symptom, and while shortness of breath may occur, it usually occurs later, after the wheezing.

Other important symptoms to monitor include postnasal drip and activity of esophageal reflux and heartburn. It's also helpful to monitor your triggers and whether you've developed a respiratory infection. If yellow-green phlegm develops, it's probably time for an antibiotic.

Shortness of breath can also be monitored, although asthma is not the only cause of this. Some people with asthma may develop shortness of breath from heart dysfunction or loss of strength in their leg muscles from the prednisone therapy. Shortness of breath might also occur when someone gains weight or is out of condition.

Special monitoring techniques are available for asthma: peak flow and the forced expired volume of air in one second, FEV_1. These can be especially helpful when someone first develops asthma.

The FEV_1 is the most accurate, although the peak flow is the most commonly used monitor. You blow into a tube and the measurement is recorded. You can color code the results in green, yellow, and use red for the danger zone. You may see a decrease before you develop symptoms so that you can use your bronchodilator inhaler early, preventing an audible asthma attack. In addition, you can write down your activities during the peak flow monitoring and might discover triggers of your asthma attacks.

When you monitor a disease you need to ask three questions. Are the symptoms better? Are they the same? Are they worse? If they're better, take no action. If wheezing or chest tightness is the same, take another puff of the bronchodilator inhaler. If they're worse, and not improving with the inhaler, especially if the symptoms worsen quickly, you might need to call 911 or visit the emergency room.

———

Heather awoke one morning with her usual boundless energy. She was excited to get to her job at the medical publishing company. She had just started editing an exciting new book. She dove into the task with her usual gusto but suddenly completely lost her energy.

"What's going on?" she asked herself. "Where's my energy?"

She soon noticed muscle aches and fatigue. She took the rest of the day off and lounged around her apartment. She had asthma for several years and noticed some increased wheezing with these symptoms, so she used her bronchodilator inhaler and continued using her corticosteroid inhaler. The symptoms stabilized, and she returned to work two days later and shrugged off her discomforts as a viral infection.

Yet the annoying symptoms continued, along with a cough and some shortness of breath, forcing her to see the doctor.

"You appear to have a mild viral pneumonia," Dr. Kory explained as they reviewed Heather's chest x-ray, which showed some hazy shadows. "Your lungs sound normal, and your blood tests are normal. So let's monitor things for awhile to see what happens."

"Sounds good to me," Heather said with relief, feeling more energized about dealing with her symptoms.

During the next 48 hours, the respiratory symptoms did not improve and might have worsened slightly, but the difference was not enough to warrant a call to Dr. Kory.

So, she monitored the symptoms for another 48 hours. This time, something happened. She developed numbness in her lips, a flushed face, and a fierce headache. She felt like it was a stroke.

"Whoa, what's going on this time? What does this have to do with the viral pneumonia?" Heather asked herself. She searched the internet for an answer.

She quickly found what she needed. She and a friend had Chinese take-out from a new restaurant around the corner from her apartment. Heather had forgotten to tell them to hold the monosodium glutamate (MSG) and developed the Chinese-food syndrome.

The internet provided her with the answer after she searched for her strange constellation of symptoms. The glutamate in the MSG is the basis for a naturally occurring neurotransmitter used in our brain and nervous system. Some people are sensitive to an external source of this seemingly innocuous chemical.

The symptoms are usually annoying and subside after a few hours, although serious symptoms may force a hurried visit to the emergency room.

As expected, Heather's strange symptoms disappeared within a few hours. In the meantime, she felt no worsening of her respiratory symptoms and continued to monitor them for another 48 hours. This time, there was improvement. After a few more days, she had a follow-up appointment with Dr. Kory.

"How are you today?"

"I'm better," Heather said enthusiastically. "I still have an occasional cough, but no shortness of breath, and my energy is beginning to return."

"Your chest x-ray shows improvement in the patchy infiltrates," Dr. Kory said. "You probably had a viral pneumonia and possibly a mild episode of BOOP."

Feeling better, but puzzled by this new term, Heather asked the expected question. "What's the funny word you used, BOOP?"

"It stands for bronchiolitis obliterans organizing pneumonia, which is inflammation that fills the small bronchiole airways and lungs with an organized inflammatory cellular pattern," Dr. Kory explained. "It sometimes occurs after a viral pneumonia. It may disappear on its own, or a brief course of anti-inflammatory steroid medication is used. You feel good. Your lungs sound normal. Your blood tests are normal. Let's continue to monitor the situation."

"Doctor, once again this sounds good to me."

The next several days brought continued improvement in Heather's cough. She returned to work full of energy and continued her Zumba fitness classes and kick boxing at her neighborhood workout facility. During her follow-up doctor's visit a month later, Heather reported resolution of her symptoms.

"Excellent, let's check your x-ray," Dr. Kory said.

"It looks great, and the infiltrates have disappeared. You're cured. You probably had a mild episode of BOOP that resolved through monitoring."

———

In some situations, the monitoring process can result in a cure, either because the natural course of the disease didn't require active treatment, or because individuals paid greater attention to their prescribed treatment, which improves compliance and more often results in a cure. Undertaking the monitoring process in a positive manner with positive expectations can also improve the desire to continue an exercise program, and increase your feeling of control.

———

Let's find out how our unlikely hero Billy is doing.

He had survived a severe asthma attack from pneumonia, and his asthma had stabilized. He continued to decrease the prednisone dose and used his corticosteroid inhaler daily. He rarely needed his bronchodilator inhaler.

Billy resumed studying for the law school entrance examination and working his two jobs. In the meantime, he had developed an excellent monitoring system that he discussed with Dr. Whitney.

"How are you doing?"

"I'm great," Billy said. "I like to use the computer, so I designed a color-coded graph to monitor my symptoms, mainly wheezing but also chest tightness, cough, and shortness of breath."

"How are you doing with the prednisone effects?" Dr. Whitney asked.

"Oh, I monitored everything," Billy answered. "I included increased appetite, weight gain, moon face, acne, bruising, blood pressure, and even blood sugar."

"That's fantastic, Billy," the doctor replied. "What happened?"

"It worked. I kept watching my monitoring program, and I had none of these side effects, and now I'm taking a small dose. My exercise program really helped."

"What about peak-flow monitoring?"

"That was also helpful," Billy said. "I downloaded the numbers into my computer chart and was surprised at the findings."

"What do you mean?"

"Look at these tracings," Billy said. "They show I have asthma attacks for three days, then nothing, and then two days, then nothing, and then another group of attacks for three days. What's going on?"

"Hmm. What did you mark down for activities?"

"Nothing unusual, just studying and working at the two jobs."

"Did you have any exposures at work that would explain these episodes?"

"No, I work in an office and reviewed any unusual exposures from cleaning solutions, plastics fumes or epoxy materials," Billy said. "There was nothing new."

"Keep monitoring the situation, and search for clues," Dr. Whitney said.

Billy was living in New Orleans and had been studying in his apartment near the Mississippi River. He enjoyed visiting the rocky bank near a French coffee and beignet restaurant. He sometimes heard a jazz saxophone player practicing under the pier. During his run along the river, he noticed ships unloading their cargo, and there appeared to be more dust coming from the unloading bins than usual. He didn't pay too much attention to it until he realized he soon had an asthma attack.

"How are you today?" Dr. Whitney asked during Billy's next follow-up visit.

"I'm doing well, but let's review my peak-flow tracings. They still have the same pattern of asthma attacks every few days. Could it have anything to do with the cargo ships?"

"What do you mean?"

"I noticed a change recently in the loading bins near the river. It appeared more dusty than usual."

"Yes, you may be on to something," Dr. Whitney said. "People with asthma can become allergic to very specific types of exposures, including rye flour used in baking. Check out the ship logs on the internet and find out what they're carrying."

Billy returned to his apartment and researched the incoming ships. Yes, ships had carried rye flour during the same days he had experienced the asthma attacks.

He and the doctor contacted the loading area. They found out that a malfunction had occurred in the ventilation system and excessive dust had been released into the air. The process was repaired and Billy's asthma attacks stopped.

"You're a genius, Dr. Whitney," Billy said.

"No, not really," the doctor said. "You made the diagnosis with your monitoring system."

———

Billy had developed an excellent monitoring system. It may be more elaborate than you need, but the idea is sound. Create a monitoring system for your asthma.

We'll conclude Billy's story after discussing information about how to create a healing environment.

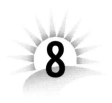

Body and Mind:
Create a Healing Environment

How can anyone with asthma say they're healed? Ask Alice. She has severe asthma. She uses her corticosteroid inhaler and long-acting bronchodilator inhaler every day. She takes brief courses of prednisone for acute asthma attacks, yet she is healed.

How can people with asthma say they are "healed" when they have an illness that requires treatment every day? Healing is within the mind. They use the power of their own words and thoughts. They use the combined energy of the mind and body.

The first four steps in the management of asthma are related to the lungs. The fifth step involves creating an environment in which to heal by combining the physical attributes of the body and the powerful influence of the mind.

There are three traditional physical components and five elements related to the mind. Let's begin with the physical components which include exercise, nutrition, and sleep.

For severe persistent asthma, a pulmonary rehabilitation program can be useful for successful management. The program can begin as soon as the asthma is stable. Your doctor writes a prescription and the office contacts a rehabilitation center at a hospital or clinic.

The program usually consists of sessions three times weekly for several weeks. You also have the option to sign up for more. The initial part of the program is a learning phase discussing asthma and talking about the best exercises for lung health. The physical phase consists of breathing exercises such as deep breathing, diaphragmatic breathing, and includes developing a strength training exercise regimen for the upper body, the core, and the lower body.

One of the benefits of pulmonary rehabilitation is that you do the exercises in a controlled environment, where your heart rate and oxygen saturation are monitored, and people are available for a safety net. An additional benefit is that you can learn how to continue the program at home or at a workout facility.

Strength training should be part of your exercise program because it can delay the loss of lean body mass. Each decade of the aging process results in loss of functional lean muscle mass, which accelerates after the age of 65. This process decreases the basal metabolic rate so fewer calories are needed; however, people usually continue to consume the same number of calories as they age, resulting in weight gain. Years of a sedentary lifestyle spent sitting at a desk can result in loss of functional lean body mass. You need to include muscle strengthening as part of your workout. A personal trainer can develop a personalized program that will not result in unwanted bulky muscles.

Short-term effects from an exercise program are felt during the first session, while long-term effects are apparent after three to six months. Full conditioning returns after about three years, at which point you will feel that you are in as good or better shape than you have ever been. Exercise is a powerful way to ignite your latent energy system, creating positive energy that can be transformed for successful management of your asthma.

Healthy nutrition is fundamental for managing your asthma, especially for people who take prednisone. Meeting with a nutritionist while going to your pulmonary rehabilitation program can be useful because of the new knowledge about body metabolism, hydration, vitamins, and minerals. The nutritionist can design a program that is best for you.

Just as it's important to understand everything that you can about asthma, it's helpful to obtain as much information as you can about nutrition. Learning about nutrition can help you manage your asthma. Read a book, listen to a CD, or visit the American Dietetic Association website. Nutritional management is an important part of creating an environment in which to heal.

There are many healthy ways to eat, but there are also unhealthy ways and plenty of hazardous weight-loss diets. Advice on how and what to eat seems to change every day. People can become overwhelmed and confused by so much conflicting scientific and anecdotal information.

A session with a nutritionist can be useful because there have been huge advances in the body's metabolic complexities. Nutritionists can design a program specifically for you, with the best types and quantities of foods. You'll determine your healthy weight, your percentage of body fat, the number of calories needed for your body type, and the optimal amount of water to consume each day.

There are some general guidelines for healthy eating. Begin by consuming an appropriate quantity of healthy, high-quality food at each meal. A major problem is eating too much. Most people have an instinctive drive to eat more than they need. The reality is that the correct portions are much smaller than people think they are; the older that people become, the less food they need. A large plate filled with food is too much.

Increases in typical portion sizes have resulted in increased caloric intake. The number of calories in many prepared processed foods has doubled or quadrupled during the past 20 years. The average muffin used to have 100 calories, but now a gigantic muffin can have 400 calories or more. It's an old concept, but paying attention to calories is still useful for maintaining a healthy weight.

A simple but useful guideline is to eat only when you're sitting at a table. Routinely eating on the run – while standing or in an elevator – is not healthy. This type of eating is usually emotionally based and is not the same as eating when you're hungry.

Another guideline is to swallow your food before taking a bite or talking. This can be helpful because it takes several minutes for your mind to register the feeling of fullness. Slowing down the eating process will prevent you from feeling stuffed, which feels bad and is not healthy.

The types of foods that you eat are important. There are good fats and bad fats, good carbohydrates and bad ones. Most proteins are good, but their sources can be bad, especially if they're bathed in saturated fat. New information is emerging daily.

Some foods are addictive, and as you would expect, they are generally not healthy. Sweet and salty foods often find their way into our daily routine. To eat just one piece or portion of these types of foods is almost impossible. The urge to consume them in large quantities can be overwhelming because they taste good, are widely available, and are likely to be familiar due to consumers' years of exposure to advertising.

In general, healthy foods have low or no saturated fats, no refined sugar, low or no sodium (salt), are nonprocessed, and contain fiber. It might take some extra time to read the food labels before you decide what to buy, but the benefits are worthwhile because you can refine your taste to enjoy naturally occurring flavors, undisturbed by numerous additives. Foods without barcodes are usually healthy, and you probably won't eat them in huge quantities. The less you eat of processed foods with a long list of ingredients, the better. The way that you eat and what you eat can have a great effect on your ability to manage disease.

Sleep is the third traditional tool that you can use to create an environment in which to heal. On the basis of years of study, eight hours of sleep appears to be a requirement for a healthy life. Most people just don't get enough sleep.

Take the five-minute sleep test. Sit in a chair in a quiet room. If you fall asleep within five minutes, you flunk the test. This might be only an isolated result, or it may mean that you are chronically sleep-deprived, which causes neural behavioral changes and cardiovascular complications. In addition, if you randomly fall asleep in five minutes, this is a potentially dangerous and unhealthy situation. You could fall asleep while with family and friends, during an important meeting at work, or even while driving.

A healthy sleep-hygiene program consists of not allowing yourself to fall asleep watching television before you go to bed, not eating or eating little within three hours before you go to bed, and going to sleep and waking up at regular times.

A brief nap in the afternoon may be effective for some individuals, but sleeping one to two hours just before you go to bed will have a devastating result. You will be awake for hours and will toss and turn throughout the night.

Sometimes a relaxation technique such as yoga or a deep-breathing exercise can be helpful before you go to bed. Sleeping pills are not needed if you have a successful sleep-hygiene program. Managing sleep successfully can have a profound influence on the creation of an environment in which to heal.

———

Using your mind can be an important part of asthma management. There are several factors to consider.

First, use a positive approach to the illness. You can manage your asthma. You are in charge of your asthma. You will take your medication regularly, exercise, and eat nutritious food.

Along with managing your asthma in a positive manner, create intense confidence in yourself. Know that you can manage the asthma with confidence. This will give you energy to succeed.

Second, use visualization. Visualize strong healthy airway cells replacing inflamed cells. Begin by visualizing one cell, then 100 cells, and then millions of healthy cells replacing the inflamed cells. You can use this mental imaging daily or whenever you think about it.

Third, have compassion for your lungs. Portions of your lungs are perfect; the asthma is the issue and can be relegated to the background. Be good to your lungs.

Fourth, use controlled breathing. If you are having an asthma attack, try diaphragmatic breathing – put your hand on your stomach, breathe out as much as you can, and push in your stomach, lowering your hand. Keep breathing out as long as you can until there is no more air, then take in a new breath and repeat this for three to five breaths every few minutes. It might help.

If you're not having an attack, use controlled breathing for a calming effect and stress release. For example, concentrate on breathing in the same amount as breathing out – 50% in and 50% out – for several minutes. Breathing opposite to your usual breathing method for a few breaths can have a calming effect. Put your hand on your stomach and breathe in. Instead of having your hand lower, make your hand move upward. Try this when you find yourself stressed or nervous. You will be calmer after a few of these opposite breaths.

Yoga breathing exercises can also be helpful. Controlled breathing can have a beneficial effect on asthma.

Fifth, persistence is fundamental for these healing techniques. They take time. Learn to use all of your brainwave activity, not just the standard 14-cycles per second beta wave frequency, but also learn to use the slower and more powerful 10-cycles per second alpha and 7-cycles per second theta brainwaves to manage the healing process. Over and over, replace negative thoughts and actions with these mind-management thoughts.

Dismay and hopelessness are powerful emotional feelings that are sometimes uncontrollable and can easily trap you because they generate sympathy for yourself and from others. Do not fight these feelings. Let them occur, but replace them with positive thoughts as quickly as possible.

The mind is weak when you have these feelings of hopelessness and despair. They must be replaced with strength, resolve, and persistence, which lead to increased energy for the healthy management of your asthma.

———

Cole was angry. He felt as if he had struggled with asthma for too long. He was angry because he had this awful problem and seeing people without asthma upset him more.

"Why me?" he asked himself over and over. "What did I do to deserve this?"

He had to take prednisone. He had gained weight, he had acne, he had bruises on his hands, and his face was puffy. He was depressed at work. He had no energy. He was angry with his doctor because the doctor couldn't cure him. He believed his doctor didn't know anything about asthma.

He wanted the doctor to make it go away. There must be someone that can do this for him.

So, he began his search.

He soon found the answer and it wasn't what he expected. Cole found out that he was the problem, not the asthma, and not the doctor. He had to take charge of the situation himself. He abandoned his negative thoughts and his anger about the asthma, about why he had asthma, and about the dreadful effects of prednisone. He began to think about positive events.

Cole realized that his asthma attacks had disappeared with prednisone treatment and the dose was being decreased. He was not wheezing. His x-ray was normal. He had learned to use his corticosteroid inhaler and knew when to use his bronchodilator inhaler. He had identified his triggers. He began to visualize healing his lungs. He had compassion for his lungs. He developed confidence in himself and his doctors.

Cole noticed a flier at work about three introductory exercise sessions with a personal trainer. He signed up for the program and was amazed when his energy returned. He soon found he was no longer thinking about the struggles with his asthma. In the meantime, he no longer had to take the prednisone.

Cole turned a struggling, frustrating, and potentially dangerous course of asthma into a management success.

———

Creating a healing environment can be a tremendously beneficial part of asthma management. Cole did the right thing.

Now, let's finish Billy's story.

———

Billy had learned all he could about asthma. He understood the diagnostic process and the treatment options. He developed a monitoring system. He was managing his asthma successfully. The final step was to create a healing environment.

"Let's talk about a pulmonary rehabilitation program," Dr. Whitney said.

"I'm too young for that," Billy said. "I don't think I need it."

"You'll be surprised," the doctor asserted. "You're already out of condition from your bad asthma attack, even though it was only a week in the hospital and several days of recovery.

A number of years ago, doctors conducted an experiment by having several healthy medical students stay in bed all day and night for six weeks. At the end of the time period, the students had become so weak and out of condition, it took them three months to return to normal strength."

"That's convincing enough for me. I'll go."

Billy attended the rehabilitation course three times each week and found it to be much more useful than he had expected. He learned more about his lungs. He also learned breathing exercises, and about an excellent group of aerobic and strengthening exercises.

"How's your nutritional program?" Dr. Whitney asked Billy during a follow-up visit.

"No idea. I eat what's available and tastes good."

"You're still taking prednisone. It'll make you eat everything in sight," the doctor said. "I'd suggest you see the nutritionist while you're at the rehabilitation program. The nutritionist is phenomenal. In the past, nutritionists designed diets for patients in hospitals. Now they know about the digestive system; carbohydrate, fat, and protein metabolism; water requirements; and calorie requirements. They know about vitamin and mineral supplements. Importantly, they understand the benefits of aerobic and strengthening exercises to prevent age-related muscle deterioration. They're anti-aging experts."

"You're right again," Billy said. "I had no idea nutritionists could help so much."

"One last thing," Dr. Whitney said. "How's your sleep program?"

"My what?"

"Your sleeping schedule?"

"That's what I thought you were talking about," Billy replied with a sigh. "I have no sleep schedule. I work two jobs every day and study all night. I sleep when I can. I sometimes find myself falling asleep while watching TV, and then I can't sleep the rest of the night."

"Prednisone is going to alter your sleep pattern, so you need to pay attention."

"What do you suggest?"

"There are several factors to consider," Dr. Whitney said. "Try not to nap or fall asleep shortly before going to bed, and no eating or snacking before going to bed. Go to bed at exactly the same time each night, and eight hours later, wake up at the same time each morning."

"That's a ton of rules."

"Yes, but they're easy to remember and easy to follow," the doctor said. "Some of them can be broken for social events and other reasons, but if you follow them most days, you'll have a huge amount of energy to do everything you want to do.

You won't flunk the sleep test – you won't fall asleep when you sit quietly for five minutes. A side benefit is that you'll find yourself less irritable, more tolerant of people's minor imperfections, and not complaining about every small annoyance throughout the day."

"Sounds good. I'll try it," Billy said.

"Now that your exercise program, a controlled nutritional program, and a good sleep plan are in place, there are a few mind-energy-related factors that can also help you manage your asthma," Dr. Whitney said.

"What are they?"

"You're doing the first one. You need a healthy approach to the disease. You get a gold star for this. You have developed an excellent attitude toward this illness. You know you can manage it, and you're learning how to do it."

"That wasn't always the case," Billy said. "I was angry and frustrated at first, but I realized that wasn't helping the situation so I decided it's better to think in a positive way toward the asthma.

"What else?"

"Visualization can help. You can visualize healthy cells replacing the inflamed airway cells."

"Sounds a little soft," Billy said. "But I guess it won't hurt."

"Good," Dr. Whitney said. "You also need intense confidence in yourself and everyone around you."

"That's easy for me now," Billy said. "Again, at first I was scared, but over time I regained my confidence, and now I know I can manage the situation."

"Another factor is to have compassion for your lungs."

"Whoa, you lost me, Doc," Billy said, bewildered. "It sounds crazy to me."

"Compassion is a great word," the doctor said.

"Some Tibetan monks live their entire lives meditating about compassion. They're amazing. People in their presence are filled with love and peace, even without talking to them or touching them. Be good to your lungs. They're perfect. Treat them well."

"Compassion is an interesting word. I'll try it."

"The last one is controlled breathing."

"You're losing me. I'm thinking in a positive manner. I'm going to use visualization. I am going to give my lungs compassion. That's enough for me."

"That's great. In addition, you can add controlled breathing exercises as many times as you wish," Dr. Whitney said.

"For people with asthma there is one helpful technique during an asthma attack, and two things you can do in between attacks."

"So, what are they?"

"For an asthma attack, you can use diaphragmatic breathing," Dr. Whitney said.

"Here's how it works. Put your hand on your stomach, and breathe out as much as you can and pushing in your stomach, lowering your hand. Stop when you run out of air and take in another breath. Do this for three to five breaths every few minutes during the asthma attack."

"Let's try it while you're sitting here."

Billy put his hand across his stomach, took in a breath, and pushed out the air as much as he could until the air stopped. Then he took in another breath, repeating it for three or four breaths.

"That's amazing," Billy said. "I think that'll really help when I'm struggling with an asthma attack.

"What are the other two techniques?" Billy asked, now excited to hear about them.

"They're reflex-based relaxing and calming techniques," Dr. Whitney said.

"The first one is equal inspiration and expiration. Breathe in the same amount of air as you breathe out for one to two minutes.

"The second one is opposite of diaphragm breathing. This time, hold your hand on your stomach, breathe in and move your hand up as you fill your abdomen with air. Use this to calm yourself and release stress if you have to give a speech or take a test."

"Sounds simple," Billy said. "Can I try the belly breathing one?"

He put his hand across his stomach and took in a deep breath. He didn't do it correctly at first, but after two or three tries, he mastered it.

"Unbelievable!" Billy exclaimed. "It makes you instantly calm."

"That's it," the doctor said. "Now you can use it whenever you need to."

"Thank you for all of your help, Dr. Whitney," Billy said. "Now I'm definitely prepared to manage the asthma and manage it well."

"You did all of the work. I just showed you how. I wish you good health and success with your asthma management."

———

Billy is a hero because he learned to manage his asthma so well that it faded from his conscious mind, freeing him to enjoy his life and be creative. He successfully completed law school and built a thriving law firm.

You can create an environment in which to heal.

Design an exercise program, a good nutritional program, and an effective sleep- hygiene program.

Use your mind. Think in a positive way toward asthma. Develop confidence in yourself and your health team.

Visualize healthy airways and lungs.

Have compassion for your lungs.

Use controlled breathing. Be persistent.

You are in charge of your asthma.

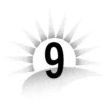

Answers to Common and Basic Questions About Asthma

We've reviewed the five steps toward asthma management. During the course of your asthma, it's helpful to continuously reevaluate these steps. New diagnostic and treatment information is disclosed every day. People with asthma and their families and friends all over the world routinely ask specific questions about asthma. Examine the list below and you might find answers to your questions.

What's asthma? Asthma is narrowing of the airways caused by underlying, persistent inflammation and bronchospasm. Asthma is an underlying tendency of your bronchial airways to constrict and narrow from a particular trigger.

Where did the word come from? The word asthma is from the Greek word that means to pant or breathe hard.

When was asthma identified? Ancient Egyptian and Greek physicians described asthmatic symptoms.

Who develops asthma? Asthma can develop at any age. Children who develop asthma most likely have allergies and a parent, often a mother, who also has asthma. For adults, it may be caused by a latent allergy or recurrence of childhood asthma, or it may be from an unknown cause, or in rare situations, from a respiratory infection or a hazardous exposure.

What are the types of asthma? They include childhood asthma, adult-onset asthma, aspirin-induced asthma, allergy asthma, exercise-induced asthma, and occupational asthma.

What's exercise-induced asthma? This can be triggered by having an increased volume of cold or dry air go through the bronchial airways which often happens during exercise.

What's occupational asthma? This is new-onset asthma induced by sensitization to a specific substance at work or recurrence of past asthma induced by exposure to an inhaled irritant at work.

What are the first symptoms of asthma? They are chest tightness and a wheezing noise during exhalation.

What is the most common physical finding? Wheezing through a stethoscope.

What does the chest x-ray show? It's usually normal, unless there is a respiratory infection or a non-asthma cause of the asthma. Then, a high-resolution chest computer tomography, or CT, scan may be helpful. The chest x-ray is normal because asthma is inflammation of the airways and not the lungs, and the airways are too thin to show up on the standard chest x-ray.

What do the pulmonary function tests show? The forced expired volume in one second, or FEV_1, is the single most important test to show asthma. This is the amount of air exhaled during the first second, and if bronchospasm is narrowing the airways, this value will be decreased. The vital capacity, which measures the amount of air in the lungs, may be normal, or if the asthma is severe, it will be decreased. The ratio of the expired volume in one second to the vital capacity, or FEV_1/FVC in percent, measures the flow of air from the lungs, and is low, especially during an asthma attack. The diffusing capacity, a measure of oxygen exchange in the lungs, is normal and may be increased in asthma because the upper lungs are utilized more in asthma. Oxygen saturation is normal but will be decreased during a severe attack.

What is a post-bronchodilator test? The FEV_1 is measured as a baseline. If asthma or reactive airway syndrome is suspected, a bronchodilator agent is given by an inhaler or nebulizer. Generally, there is no change, but a 12% or more increase indicates asthma if there are appropriate corresponding symptoms.

What is an inhalation challenge test? This determines whether the airways react to certain types of challenges such as methacholine, exercise, cold air, and a potential toxic occupational or environmental exposure. Methacholine is a substance that is opposite of a bronchodilator agent. It constricts the airways in susceptible people. This test is performed if someone has unusual symptoms and normal pulmonary function tests to see if they have reactive airways or asthma. The baseline FEV_1 test is obtained. A very small methacholine dose is given and the FEV_1 is obtained again. This is repeated three or four more times with increasing doses. If the FEV_1 decreases by 20%, it is a positive test and the process is stopped. If there is no decrease, it is a negative test. Exercise, cold air or workplace exposure material can be substituted for the methacholine. A 20% decrease in FEV_1 is a positive test.

What do blood tests show? Most blood tests will be normal. The white blood cell, or WBC, analysis might show increased eosinophils, which are white cells containing red granules, and suggests allergy asthma. Usually 1% to 3% eosinophils are detected. There may be 10% to 15% eosinophils with allergic asthma.

What is allergy testing? There are two types. Skin testing is the typical type, which means that a small amount of the allergen, such as tree pollen or grass is placed on the skin. The test is negative if nothing happens; or if it's red, it's graded on a mild, moderate, or severe degree. IgE immune blood testing is the other type, which measures the immune response to various agents such as bee stings or peanuts.

What is the natural history of asthma, or what is the outcome over time for asthma that is not treated? It depends on the category. Mild intermittent asthma treated with an occasional use of a bronchodilator may occur over a lifetime or it could disappear after several years. Severe persistent asthma would have a poor outcome without active treatment. For some individuals, this severe type of asthma is variable over time, with intense severity for several months or years followed by cycles of less intensity. The good news is that asthma is treatable and people can manage their asthma successfully.

What are the treatment options? Treatment depends on the severity classification, and sometimes on the type of asthma. Intermittent use of a bronchodilator inhaler for wheezing or chest tightness is the best treatment for mild intermittent asthma and for exercise-induced asthma. The addition of a corticosteroid inhaler is used for mild persistent asthma. For moderate persistent asthma, a long-acting bronchodilator inhaler is used along with the steroid inhaler. For severe persistent allergy asthma, treatments can address the underlying allergic nature of the asthma. For others with severe persistent asthma, prednisone tablets might be needed in addition to the inhaled steroid and a bronchodilator.

What are the side effects of prednisone and how can they be managed? The potential side effects are numerous and vary from person to person. Some individuals have no side effects, and others may have multiple adverse reactions. Most are reversible, but some are not. It's important to read the package insert for details.

An increased appetite and overwhelming desire to eat is the first effect of prednisone. This can be managed by staying to a routine of eating small portions in a regular manner. Weight gain is related to the first effect and is managed through eating small portions of healthy foods.

Other effects include the development of a "moon face" or "cushingoid" appearance. Steroid "fat pads" might develop on the chest below the chin and at the base of the back of the neck. Purplish-red blotches and bruises might appear on the skin of the hands and arms from fragile capillaries. Softening of the bones and osteoporosis might occur that can be managed by calcium, one of the biphosphonates, and exercise. Diabetes might occur in individuals with borderline diabetes, and hypertension might occur. Both of these effects can be treated with diabetic or hypertension medications, if necessary.

Lower extremity fluid retention might occur, which can be treated with a diuretic, if necessary. Proximal muscle weakness might occur. Psychological effects such as euphoria and high energy as well as depression and disorientation might occur.

Two effects that are not reversible include cataracts and aseptic necrosis of the hip. Eye surgery may be required for the cataracts and hip replacement may be needed for the aseptic necrosis. Maintaining a healthy weight may decrease the risk of developing aseptic necrosis.

Long-term prednisone use increases the risk of bacterial and fungal infections. Antibiotics and anti-fungal medications, sometimes intravenously, are needed to treat these infections. *Pneumocystis*, a small parasitic organism, could develop, and Bactrim® would be given three times weekly as prevention. Individuals with a past tuberculous infection and positive TB test are at risk of developing active tuberculosis so isoniazid, or INH, tablets may be given.

Withdrawal side effects may also occur as the prednisone is decreased, especially after prednisone has been taken for more than a year. These effects include muscle aches, fatigue, weakness, and transient depression.

The side effects lessen when 7.5 mg or less of the medication is given because this is the amount of prednisone made daily by the adrenal glands.

How do I monitor my asthma? You can monitor your symptoms. Wheezing is the most common and sometimes chest tightness may be an early symptom. Some people with asthma have a cough too. The peak flow measurement or the forced expired volume in one second, or

FEV_1, can be monitored to identify early changes and identify asthma triggers.

How can I create a healing environment? A pulmonary rehabilitation program and a home exercise program can initiate the healing process. A good nutritional program can also be helpful by managing right-size portions of healthy, high-quality foods with low amounts of sodium, sugar, saturated fats, and proper amounts of fiber.

Use controlled breathing exercises such as breathing in the same amount of air as breathing out for several minutes, and using the opposite breathing technique by moving the stomach out while breathing in for one minute. Use diaphragmatic breathing during an asthma attack – by blowing out as much air as possible while moving your hand on your stomach downward.

Use the power of your mind during the healing process. Approach your management of asthma in a positive manner. You can manage your asthma. Visualize replacing inflamed airway cells with lively, healthy cells. Develop a deep confidence in the ability of your body to heal and restore health. Have compassion for your lungs and treat them well. Persist with these concepts, and they'll become a part of you.

Is asthma contagious? No. Asthma is inflammation of the bronchial airways, and is not caused by a microbe that can infect other people.

Is asthma inherited? Asthma occurs in family members and some twins have had asthma. The specific genes have not been discovered. Children with asthma tend to have mothers with asthma.

Does smoking cause asthma? Smoking may not cause typical asthma; however, smoking may cause respiratory bronchiolitis, which is inflammation of the small bronchioles entering the lungs, and may cause increased airway reactivity. The thousands of chemicals and particles in cigarette smoke will cause inflammation of the airways, resulting in ongoing continual inflammation and bronchospasm. In a nonsmoker, cigarette smoke can trigger an asthma attack, especially in an enclosed room.

Can asthma be cured? No, but asthma can be managed and controlled with appropriate treatment. The natural history of some types of asthma consists of periods of quiescence, sometimes for several years, and it may resolve over time in some individuals. There are people, however, who develop permanent scarring around their bronchial airways.

Can people die from asthma? Yes, a person can die from a severe asthma attack. A severe attack may occur at any age, in both men and women, and generally only in individuals with moderate or severe persistent asthma. The risk factors include neglecting daily inhaled steroids and relying solely on rescue bronchodilators, and not knowing triggers. Also, a person who has a severe asthma attack might have ignored the signs that had been coming on for hours or days, until it had become irreversible.

Are there "alternative medicine" treatments for asthma? So far, bronchodilator and steroid inhalers are the best treatments. Other treatments have not been found to have consistent results. Creating an environment for healing can include pulmonary rehabilitation, an exercise program, a healthy nutrition program, a good sleep-hygiene program, and some mind-body techniques.

Are there any new treatments for asthma? Xolair® helps some individuals with allergic asthma by blocking the body's ability to produce an allergic reaction when an allergen is present. A new therapy called bronchial thermoplasty is when a bronchoscope is used to produce high heat energy to destroy the excessive smooth muscle tissue in the asthma bronchial airways, and it is used three times every three weeks. This therapy has been approved by the FDA and it seems to be reducing attacks while maintaining lung function.

What are the challenges for treating asthma globally? From the standpoint of public policy, the unequal distribution of healthcare availability between high- and low-income people continues to be a challenge. Although inhaled steroids do not cost as much as IgE inhibitors, their cost can be significant for individuals with low incomes, so many go without and end up in an emergency room.

For people who can afford their medications, the challenge is for them to take them on a regular prescribed basis and maintain their asthma action plans.

What type of exercises can I do with asthma? Any type of exercise is beneficial. The best one is the one that you enjoy. One good approach is to participate in a pulmonary rehabilitation program three times weekly for ten weeks. You will be taught specific breathing exercises for asthma and learn an exercise program that you can do at home or at a workout center near your home. Walking, swimming, bicycling, and aerobic dances are all good forms of exercise. You can also go to a workout center where personal trainers can teach you an exercise routine with the equipment such as a treadmill, stationary bicycle, elliptical machine, rowing machine, and light free weights.

Muscle strengthening exercises are important to prevent loss of functional lean body mass. The exercises are designed to tone the upper-body muscles, the core abdominal back muscles, and the lower extremity muscles. The exercise program is not only helpful for the management of asthma, but also management of the prednisone's side effects.

Will yoga help asthma? Yoga can be beneficial. Other exercise such as tai chi and qigong can be beneficial.

Is a pulmonary rehabilitation program helpful? It's very helpful, and it can begin as soon as the symptoms begin to improve. Part of the program involves learning about your lungs and doing breathing exercises. The other part of the program is to exercise and develop a home exercise program. Exercise will improve muscle oxygen efficiency and conditioning, and it will also provide a sense of well being.

I'm short of breath when I exercise. What can I do? This depends on whether the shortness of breath is due to asthma or the more likely reason, poorly conditioned muscles. Taking the pulmonary rehabilitation program in a controlled environment with oximeter monitoring will allow you to push yourself to gain muscle conditioning, but not so much that you will develop cardiorespiratory dysfunction.

I'm angry about having asthma. Is there anything I can do? Being upset is a natural reaction. "Why me? Why did I get asthma? What did I do to deserve this?" Asthma can occur at any time in anyone in the world. Being frightened is also a natural feeling that can be managed. Approach the asthma in a positive manner. The body has a powerful ability to heal. You can manage your disease.

I don't think my doctor knows anything about asthma. What can I do? Most family physicians and primary care doctors are current when it comes to the diagnosis and treatment of asthma. If your questions about the diagnosis and treatment options are answered to your satisfaction, and you are able to manage your asthma without it interfering with your life, you are likely in good hands.

If your questions are not answered, and if you're confused about the diagnosis and the management plan, you can seek an additional evaluation.

How do I get back my lung capacity? An exercise program is the best way to gain strength and energy.

———

Asthma management is up to you. You now have a five-step approach.

Learn everything you can about asthma and continue that learning.

Understand the diagnostic process because asthma is recurrent and you need to know how to determine whether it's asthma or something else.

Knowing the treatment options is an ongoing process as new developments continue to occur.

Monitor your asthma because the ongoing information will lead to successful management. Continue to create an environment in which to heal using the mind-body connections.

You are in charge. Manage your asthma.

You can do this better than anyone else.

Your chances of success are unlimited.

About the Author

Dr. Gary Epler is a clinician, author, and educator. He has written the critically-acclaimed personalized health book, *You're the Boss: Manage Your Disease.* Dr. Epler obtained his medical degree from Tulane University in New Orleans and his master's in public health from Harvard University in Boston. Recognized yearly from 1994 to 2011 in *The Best Doctors in America*, Dr. Gary Epler is a pulmonary consultant at the Brigham and Women's Hospital and Dana-Farber Cancer Institute as well as a clinical associate professor of medicine at Harvard Medical School. For 15 years, he chaired the Department of Medicine at New England Baptist Hospital in Boston.

While exploring Colombia and the Amazon jungle as a medical student, Dr. Epler discovered the missing cercaria stage of the lung fluke. Later, he probed the nutritional needs of people living in the lower Sahara region of Africa, and he managed the tuberculosis refugee program in Southeast Asia.

Dr. Epler is world-renowned for describing the lung disorder bronchiolitis obliterans organizing pneumonia, or BOOP, which spurred international research and study. In the 1990s, he developed an interactive website about BOOP, idiopathic pulmonary fibrosis, or IPF, and sarcoidosis for patients and their families.

In addition to his clinical and research work, Dr. Epler strives to educate. He became editor-in-chief of an internet-based educational program in critical care and pulmonary medicine, offered by the American College of Chest Physicians. *Business Week* acclaimed him for his development of e-health educational programs that enable patients to manage their health and diseases.

Dr. Epler was recognized as one of *Boston Magazine's* "2007 Top Doctors in Town." He has received numerous teaching awards. He has published books about occupational lung diseases and bronchiolar diseases. He has written more than 100 scientific articles and presented some 350 lectures and seminars worldwide. He is a frequent guest on radio and television shows.

Active in his community, Dr. Epler has coached soccer, hockey, and basketball, and recently coached a college-club baseball team. He lives near Boston with his wife Joan and his two sons.

Visit www.eplerhealth.com for ongoing information about personalized health and to help manage your asthma.

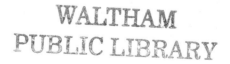